Ovarian Cancer Screening

Special Issue Editor
Edward J. Pavlik

MDPI • Basel • Beijing • Wuhan • Barcelona • Belgrade

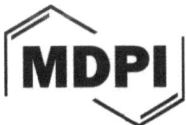

MDPI

Special Issue Editor
Edward J. Pavlik
University of Kentucky College of Medicine
USA

Editorial Office
MDPI AG
St. Alban-Anlage 66
Basel, Switzerland

This edition is a reprint of the Special Issue published online in the open access journal *Diagnostics* (ISSN 2075-4418) in 2017 (available at: http://www.mdpi.com/journal/diagnostics/special_issues/ovarian_cancer).

For citation purposes, cite each article independently as indicated on the article page online and as indicated below:

Lastname, F.M.; Lastname, F.M. Article title. *Journal Name*. **Year**. *Article number*, page range.

First Edition 2018

Image courtesy of Tom Dolan and Edward J. Pavlik

ISBN 978-3-03842-716-2 (Pbk)
ISBN 978-3-03842-715-5 (PDF)

Table of Contents

About the Special Issue Editor

Edward J. Pavlik, Professor, I serve on the editorial board of seven journals with service that also includes reviewing in 2017 for the United States Preventive Health Task Force. In 2016–2017, I completed 74 journal reviewing requests. I am an invited expert to the American Institute of Ultrasound in Medicine (AIUM). On a monthly basis, I provide a compilation of publications related to the field of gynecologic oncology from scholarly journals for the International Gynecologic Cancer Society (IGCS) of which I am a member. This compilation is called In The Know—Eds List of Gyn Onc Literature of Significance and is at https://igcs.org/in-the-know/. I have published over 100 papers in refereed journals, and have seven contributions to books, including two as editor. I have fourteen publications that have received over 100 citations, 62 cited at least 10 times and a total of more than 4300 citations of my publications as determined by Google Scholar.

diagnostics

MDPI

Editorial

Ovarian Cancer Screening:
Lessons about Effectiveness

Edward J. Pavlik

Division of Gynecologic Oncology, Department of Obstetrics and Gynecology, University of Kentucky Chandler Medical Center-Markey Cancer Center, Lexington, KY 40536, USA; Epaul1@uky.edu

Received: 18 December 2017; Accepted: 29 December 2017; Published: 29 December 2017

Ovarian cancer screening has been described in scientific reports [1–4], as well as in reviews and summaries. Scientific reports contain the facts of a study, while reviews and summaries present interpretations. Presented here are scientific reports which add considerable information to the area of early stage ovarian cancer detection and the application of this detection to ovarian cancer screening. In the present reports:

Froyman and collaborators have assessed and compared the performance of different ultrasound-based International Ovarian Tumor Analysis (IOTA) strategies and subjective assessment for the diagnosis of early stage ovarian malignancy. This important study establishes that the approaches that are taken present a good discrimination between early stage ovarian malignancy and benign abnormalities of the ovary [5].

Baldwin and co-investigators have realized that oophorectomy confers protection against ovarian cancer to the population that has undergone this surgical procedure. As a consequence, risk estimates of ovarian cancer must be adjusted for this protection so that true risk is not underestimated. When these adjustments were made, the rates of ovarian cancer were substantially higher when salpingo-oophorectomy was considered [6].

Ore and associates have examined how frequently and confidently healthy women report symptoms during surveillance for ovarian cancer. They found that the frequency of symptoms relevant to ovarian cancer was more than two hundred times higher than the occurrence of ovarian cancer and that 80.1% of women expressed confidence in the symptoms they reported [7].

Miller and her investigational team compared complications of surgical intervention for participants in the Kentucky Ovarian Cancer Screening Program to results from the Prostate, Lung, Colorectal, and Ovarian Cancer Screening trial (PLCO). They report that complications resulting from surgery performed in the Kentucky Ovarian Cancer Screening Program were infrequent and significantly fewer than reported in the Prostate, Lung, Colorectal and Ovarian Cancer Screening trial. Complications observed were mostly minor (93%) and were more common in cancer versus non-cancer surgery [8].

Ormsby and collaborators present arguments in favor of serial ultrasonography as an alternative to immediate surgery so that any benign abnormality will have the opportunity to resolve. Ultimately, this report presents arguments relative to the benefits of surveillance [9].

Ed Pavlik presents ten critical considerations for ovarian cancer screening, some of which have not been realized in published ovarian screening study reports. These considerations are presented in depth along with illustrations of how they impact the outcomes of ovarian cancer screening trials. These considerations highlight effects that have an important bearing on ovarian screening outcomes and their interpretations [10].

Michael Andrykowski presents considerations that have psychological and behavioral impacts on individuals participating in ovarian screening. His findings suggest that a "normal" screening test result can have psychological benefits, including increased positive affect and beliefs in the efficacy of screening. Moreover, any psychological or behavioral harms attributable to ovarian cancer screening are generally very modest in severity and duration, and might be counterbalanced by psychological benefits accruing to women who participate in routine ovarian cancer screening and receive normal test results [11].

Koshiyama and collaborators present current issues that are related to ovarian cancer and screening. They report that the efficacy of ovarian cancer screening may be higher in Asia than in Europe and the USA. These investigators review the re-analysis of PLCO screening data when cancers presenting more than one year after screening are excluded and show a significant survival benefit in the PLCO screening. They highlight their views by considering the difficulties of detecting Type II ovarian carcinomas [12].

Chris Smith examines the effects that ovarian cancer has on patients and their families. The rigors of treatment conspire with the inevitability of recurrence in the eyes of this first year resident in Obstetrics and Gynecology. He postulates that in the absence of effective therapies, early detection holds the greatest promise [13].

Fred Ueland relates the 50 year history of biomarkers and ultrasound in the context of ovarian cancer. He emphasizes the serial application of both biomarkers and ultrasound. Importantly, he looks to what the future may bring with regard to the utilization of biomarkers and ultrasound in routine patient exams [14].

Taken together, these authors have provided both original data and overviews of ovarian cancer screening studies that enhance the present interpretation of this type of screening.

Conflicts of Interest: The author declares no conflict of interest.

References

1. Kobayashi, H.; Yamada, Y.; Sado, T.; Sakata, M.; Yoshida, S.; Kawaguchi, R.; Kanayama, S.; Shigetomi, H.; Haruta, S.; Tsuji, Y.; et al. A randomized study of screening for ovarian cancer: A multicenter study in Japan. *Int. J. Gynecol. Cancer* **2008**, *18*, 414–420. [CrossRef] [PubMed]
2. Pavlik, E.J.; Ueland, F.R.; Miller, R.W.; Ubellacker, J.M.; Desimone, C.P.; Elder, J.; Hoff, J.; Baldwin, L.; Kryscio, R.J.; Nagell, J.R., Jr. Frequency and disposition of ovarian abnormalities followed with serial transvaginal ultrasonography. *Obstet. Gynecol.* **2013**, *122*, 210–217. [CrossRef] [PubMed]
3. Buys, S.S.; Partridge, E.; Black, A.; Johnson, C.C.; Lamerato, L.; Isaacs, C.; Reding, D.J.; Greenlee, R.T.; Yokochi, L.A.; Kessel, B.; et al. Effect of screening on ovarian cancer mortality—The Prostate, Lung, Colorectal and Ovarian (PLCO) Cancer Screening Randomized Controlled Trial. *JAMA* **2011**, *305*, 2295–2303. [CrossRef] [PubMed]
4. Jacobs, I.J.; Menon, U.; Ryan, A.; Gentry-Maharaj, A.; Burnell, M.; Kalsi, J.K.; Amso, N.N.; Apostolidou, S.; Benjamin, E.; Cruickshank, D.; et al. Ovarian cancer screening and mortality in the UK Collaborative Trial of Ovarian Cancer Screening (UKCTOCS): A randomised controlled trial. *Lancet* **2016**, *387*, 945–956. [CrossRef]
5. Froyman, W.; Wynants, L.; Landolfo, C.; Bourne, T.; Valentin, L.; Testa, A.; Sladkevicius, P.; Franchi, D.; Fischerova, D.; Savelli, L.; et al. Validation of the Performance of International Ovarian Tumor Analysis (IOTA) Methods in the Diagnosis of Early Stage Ovarian Cancer in a Non-Screening Population. *Diagnostics* **2017**, *7*, 32. [CrossRef] [PubMed]
6. Baldwin, L.A.; Chen, Q.; Tucker, T.C.; White, C.G.; Ore, R.N.; Huang, B. Ovarian Cancer Incidence Corrected for Oophorectomy. *Diagnostics* **2017**, *7*, 19. [CrossRef] [PubMed]
7. Ore, R.M.; Baldwin, L.; Woolum, D.; Elliott, E.; Wijers, C.; Chen, C.-Y.; Miller, R.W.; DeSimone, C.P.; Ueland, F.R.; Kryscio, R.J.; et al. Symptoms Relevant to Surveillance for Ovarian Cancer. *Diagnostics* **2017**, *7*, 18. [CrossRef] [PubMed]
8. Baldwin, L.A.; Pavlik, E.J.; Ueland, E.; Brown, H.E.; Ladd, K.M.; Huang, B.; DeSimone, C.P.; van Nagell, J.R.; Ueland, F.R.; Miller, R.W. Complications from Surgeries Related to Ovarian Cancer Screening. *Diagnostics* **2017**, *7*, 16. [CrossRef] [PubMed]
9. Ormsby, E.L.; Pavlik, E.J.; McGahan, J.P. Ultrasound Monitoring of Extant Adnexal Masses in the Era of Type 1 and Type 2 Ovarian Cancers: Lessons Learned From Ovarian Cancer Screening Trials. *Diagnostics* **2017**, *7*, 25. [CrossRef] [PubMed]

10. Pavlik, E.J. Ten Important Considerations for Ovarian Cancer Screening. *Diagnostics* **2017**, *7*, 22. [CrossRef] [PubMed]
11. Andrykowski, M.A. Psychological and Behavioral Impact of Participation in Ovarian Cancer Screening. *Diagnostics* **2017**, *7*, 15. [CrossRef] [PubMed]
12. Koshiyama, M.; Matsumura, N.; Konishi, I. Subtypes of Ovarian Cancer and Ovarian Cancer Screening. *Diagnostics* **2017**, *7*, 12. [CrossRef] [PubMed]
13. Smith, C.G. A Resident's Perspective of Ovarian Cancer. *Diagnostics* **2017**, *7*, 24. [CrossRef] [PubMed]
14. Ueland, F.R. A Perspective on Ovarian Cancer Biomarkers: Past, Present and Yet-To-Come. *Diagnostics* **2017**, *7*, 14. [CrossRef] [PubMed]

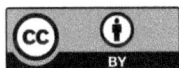

diagnostics

MDPI

Review

Subtypes of Ovarian Cancer and Ovarian Cancer Screening

Masafumi Koshiyama [1,2,*], **Noriomi Matsumura** [1] **and Ikuo Konishi** [1,3]

1   Department of Gynecology and Obstetrics, Kyoto University, Graduate School of Medicine, Sakyo-ku, Kyoto 606-8507, Japan; noriomi@kuhp.kyoto-u.ac.jp (N.M.); konishi@kuhp.kyoto-u.ac.jp (I.K.)
2   Department of Women's Health, Graduate School of Human Nursing, The University of Shiga Prefecture, 2500 Hassakacho, Hikone, Shiga 522-8533, Japan
3   Department of Obstetrics and Gynecology, National Hospital Organization Kyoto Medical Center, Fushimi-ku, Kyoto 612-8555, Japan
*   Correspondence: koshiyamam@nifty.com; Tel.: +81-749-28-8664; Fax: +81-749-28-9532

Academic Editor: Edward J. Pavlik
Received: 27 December 2016; Accepted: 27 February 2017; Published: 2 March 2017

Abstract: Ovarian cancer is the foremost cause of gynecological cancer death in the developed world, as it is usually diagnosed at an advanced stage. In this paper we discuss current issues, the efficacy and problems associated with ovarian cancer screening, and compare the characteristics of ovarian cancer subtypes. There are two types of ovarian cancer: Type I carcinomas, which are slow-growing, indolent neoplasms thought to arise from a precursor lesion, which are relatively common in Asia; and Type II carcinomas, which are clinically aggressive neoplasms that can develop de novo from serous tubal intraepithelial carcinomas (STIC) and/or ovarian surface epithelium and are common in Europe and the USA. One of the most famous studies on the subject reported that annual screening using CA125/transvaginal sonography (TVS) did not reduce the ovarian cancer mortality rate in the USA. In contrast, a recent study in the UK showed an overall average mortality reduction of 20% in the screening group. Another two studies further reported that the screening was associated with decreased stage at detection. Theoretically, annual screening using CA125/TVS could easily detect precursor lesions and could be more effective in Asia than in Europe and the USA. The detection of Type II ovarian carcinoma at an early stage remains an unresolved issue. The resolving power of CA125 or TVS screening alone is unlikely to be successful at resolving STICs. Biomarkers for the early detection of Type II carcinomas such as STICs need to be developed.

Keywords: subtypes; two types of ovarian cancer; ovarian cancer screening; CA125; transvaginal sonography

1. Introduction

Ovarian cancer is the foremost cause of gynecological cancer death and is overall one of the most frequent causes of fatal malignancy in women [1]. The symptoms are often nonspecific, hampering early detection, so the majority of patients present with advanced-stage disease.

Screening is defined as the application of a test or a combination of tests to an asymptomatic at-risk population to detect a disease at an earlier and more curable stage. In 2011, an examination of a screening program for prostate, lung, colorectal, and ovarian cancer (PLCO) in the USA revealed that annual screening using CA125/transvaginal sonography (TVS) did not markedly reduce the ovarian cancer mortality rate [2,3]. While this finding suggests that it is not possible to detect ovarian cancer at an earlier curable stage, it is possible to question the validity of these data.

Recently, the characteristics of several subtypes of ovarian cancer have been elucidated by the findings from histopathological, molecular, and genetic studies. Ovarian cancer can be roughly divided into two broad categories: Type I, in which precursor lesions in the ovaries have clearly been described; and Type II, in which such lesions have not been clearly described and tumors may develop de novo from the tubal and/or ovarian surface epithelium [4]. Understanding these characteristics is important in the effort to reduce ovarian cancer mortality.

This study first describes the characteristics of the subtypes of ovarian cancer and the results of several large-scale studies of ovarian cancer screening. We discuss current issues, the efficacy and problems associated with ovarian cancer screening, and make comparisons of the characteristics of ovarian cancer subtypes.

2. Ovarian Carcinoma Types

2.1. Type I Carcinoma

Type I carcinomas are generally slow-growing indolent neoplasms, and their precursor lesions in the ovaries have been clearly described [4].

2.1.1. Endometrioid Carcinoma and Clear Cell Carcinoma

Clear cell and endometrioid carcinomas are believed to arise from endometriosis of the ovary. Among malignant transformation cases of endometriotic cyst, serial transvaginal ultrasonography (USG) examinations revealed an increase in the cyst size [5]. Increased risks of ovarian carcinoma arising from endometriosis were associated with infertility, early menarche, and late menopause [6]. Pathologically, the co-existence of ovarian carcinoma and endometriosis is frequently observed, and in such cases endometriosis is called "atypical endometriosis", a putative precursor lesion including atypia of the cell nucleus [7].

Carcinogenesis of endometrioid and clear cell carcinomas arising from endometriotic cysts is significantly influenced by the microenvironment in the precursors [8]. The content of an endometriotic cyst (including free iron in old blood) is thought to be associated with cancer development through the induction of persistent oxidative stress [9]. The epithelial cells in the cyst are exposed to oxidative stress and hypoxia. Thus, they are subject to increased cellular and DNA damage, have less efficient DNA repair, and are easily transformed [10,11].

Somatic mutations in the ARID1A tumor-suppressor gene have been frequently identified in clear cell carcinoma. BAF250a encoded by ARID1A is a member of the SWItch/sucrose nonfermentable (SWI/SNF) complex. We recently reported that clear cell carcinomas exhibiting the loss of one or multiple SWI/SNF complex subunits demonstrated aggressive behaviors and poor prognosis [12].

2.1.2. Mucinous Carcinoma

A subset of mucinous carcinomas is thought to develop in association with ovarian benign teratomas; however, the majority of mucinous carcinomas do not show any teratomatous components [13,14]. Other theories of an ontogeny include origin from mucinous metaplasia of surface epithelial inclusions, endometriosis, and Brenner tumors [5,14]; however, these observations are relatively uncommon, except for Müllerian endocervical mucinous or mixed borderline tumors [15,16].

Morphological transitions from cystadenoma to a mucinous borderline tumor (MBT) to intraepithelial carcinoma and invasive carcinoma have occasionally been observed [17]. An increasing frequency of KRAS mutations at codons 12 and 13 has been reported in cystadenomas, MBTs, and mucinous carcinomas [18–21]. These findings support the hypothesis of the "mucinous adenoma–carcinoma sequence" [17,22] and the view that mucinous carcinomas may develop in a step-wise fashion from mucinous cystadenomas and MBTs.

2.1.3. Low-Grade Serous Carcinoma

Low-grade serous carcinomas are very rare tumors. They are genetically stable and are characterized by their low number of genetic mutations; therefore, they develop slowly from the precursors and behave in an indolent fashion. They are also thought to grow in a step-wise fashion from benign serous cystadenoma to serous borderline tumors (SBTs), and then to low-grade serous carcinoma.

p53 mutations are uncommon in low-grade serous carcinoma [23]. These carcinomas have a DNA content and level of copy number alterations that closely resembles that of SBTs [24,25].

One theory of the origin of these tumors is that they are derived from ovarian epithelial inclusions that have undergone Müllerian metaplasia [26]. The exposure of the mesothelial cells to the ovarian stromal microenvironment may result in transformation to Müllerian epithelium.

Another theory is that serous tumors may be derived from a secondary Müllerian system, arising from the embryological remnants of the proximal Müllerian ducts located within the ovarian hilm [27,28]. However, a new theory suggests that low-grade serous carcinoma may be derived from the fallopian tube. The premise is that shed tubal epithelial cells can implant on the ovarian surface epithelium, followed by the formation of inclusion cysts and transforming serous carcinoma [29,30].

2.2. Type II Carcinoma

Type II carcinomas are clinically aggressive neoplasms and may develop de novo from the tubal and/or ovarian surface epithelium.

High-Grade Serous Carcinoma

High-grade serous carcinomas account for 68% of ovarian cancer and have the worst prognosis, as they are high-grade clinically aggressive neoplasms that are usually diagnosed at an advanced stage. They show TP53 gene mutations in nearly 80% of cases [31–34] and have a high Ki67 proliferation index (50%–75%). Chromosomal rearrangements are common and associated with gene instability. Mutations in the *BRCA* 1 and 2 genes are associated with 90% of hereditary high-grade serous carcinoma cases [35].

Recently, analyses of gene expression microarray data from The Cancer Genome Atlas (TCGA) project have revealed that high-grade serous carcinoma can be classified into one of four gene expression subtypes: mesenchymal, immunoreactive, proliferative, and differentiated [36,37]. Our group reported that the progression-free and overall survival were best in the immunoreactive group, whereas the overall survival was worst in the mesenchymal transition group ($p < 0.001$ for each) [38]. Expression of vascular endothelial growth factor (VEGF) inhibits tumor immunity through the accumulation of myeloid-derived suppressor cells, and contributes to poor prognosis [39].

These tumors may develop de novo from the tubal and/or ovarian surface epithelium. In 2001, Piek et al. [40] found new transformations from hyperplastic to dysplastic lesions on tubal segments removed from women who had either *BRCA* mutations or a strong family history of ovarian carcinoma and underwent a risk-reducing bilateral salpingo-oophorectomy (BSO). These dysplastic lesions within the tubal epithelium are termed "serous tubal intraepithelial carcinomas" (STIC) and microscopic disease.

A very early abnormality termed "secretory cell outgrowths" (SCOUTs) was recently reported in tubal epithelia [41]. The TP53 signatures were the next earliest entities, and have an immunohistochemical definition of "p53-positive with a low proliferative index (Ki67 < 10%)". Developing later were "serous tubal intraepithelial lesions" (STILs) [42], also known as "transitional intraepithelial lesions of the tube" (TILTs) by some authors. These have proliferative p53 signatures, tubal dysplasia, and even tubal epithelial atypia [40,43]. Lastly, these turned into STICs; thus, STICs appear to be associated with the development of serous carcinoma.

It was recently reported that the junction of the fallopian tube epithelium with the mesothelium of the tubal serosa might be a potential site for carcinogenesis [44]. Carcinomas arising from this junctional zone can easily invade the extensive lymphovascular system under the tubal epithelium and rapidly spread throughout the abdominal cavity.

In contrast, ovarian hilum cells have shown increased transformation potential after the inactivation of tumor suppressor genes transformation-related protein 53 (Trp53) and retinoblastoma 1 (Rb1) in mice [45]. These stem cells may also be the origin of high-grade serous carcinoma.

3. Large-Scale Studies of Ovarian Cancer Screening

Ovarian cancer screening was once thought to be ineffective, but has recently been reported to result in a better prognosis than without screening [46].

3.1. A Screening Program for Prostate, Lung, Colorectal, and Ovarian Cancer

One large-scale study of ovarian cancer screening examined a screening program for prostate, lung, colorectal, and ovarian cancer (PLCO) in the USA, performed using a randomized controlled trial (RCT) [2,3]. The annual screening in this study was performed by transvaginal sonography and CA125 level measurements.

The PLCO screening arm involved 78,216 women receiving either annual screening (n = 39,105) or the usual care (n = 39,111). Ovarian cancer was diagnosed in 212 patients (0.54%) in the screening group and 176 patients (0.45%) in the standard care group. The stage distribution in the screening group was as follows: 32 (15%) cases of Stage I disease, 15 (7%) cases of Stage II disease, 120 (57%) cases of Stage III disease, and 43 (20%) cases of Stage IV disease, indicating that 77% of patients had cancer at Stage III or higher. The distribution of cancer histologies included 116 (80%) cases of serous carcinomas, five (3%) cases of mucinous carcinomas, 19 (13%) cases of endometrioid carcinomas, and six (4%) cases of clear cell carcinomas, indicating that most cases involved serous cancers.

The authors concluded that annual screening did not reduce the ovarian cancer mortality rate compared with standard care. Based on this report, ovarian cancer screening is not considered to be effective.

3.2. Re-Analysis of the PLCO Screening Data

We obtained the authors' datasets and performed a new analysis. We divided the patients who were diagnosed with ovarian cancer into two groups. One group included 101 patients whose ovarian cancers were detected through annual screening (CA125 and/or TVS) or within one year after screening. The other group included 344 patients in the screening group whose ovarian cancers were found at more than one year after screening due to the patient experiencing symptoms, as well as patients in the no screening and control groups. We previously reported these results [47]. The prognosis was significantly better in the patients in the former group than in those in the latter group (median survival: 6.1 vs. 3.3 years, p = 0.0017). Additionally, the first group contained significantly fewer Stage IV cases than the second group (13% vs. 29%, respectively, p = 0.005).

We identified two weaknesses in the PLCO screening: the group undergoing annual screening included many women who never received screening, and many patients with ovarian cancer in the screening group were diagnosed incidentally more than one year after screening, and as such could not be related to the direct effect of screening.

3.3. The United Kingdom Collaborative Trial of Ovarian Cancer Screening

The United Kingdom Collaborative Trial of Ovarian Cancer Screening (UKCTOCS) is an RCT of 202,638 women (control: 101,359; multimodal screening (MMS): 50,640; TVS alone: 50,639) [48–50]. The MMS protocol included annual CA125 screening interpreted using a patented "Risk of Ovarian Cancer" algorithm (ROCA) with TVS as a second-line test [51,52]. Ovarian cancer was diagnosed in 38 (0.08%) patients in the MMS group and 32 (0.06%) patients in the TVS group. The distribution of the cancer histologies was similar to that of the PLCO group. The distribution of the cancer stages in the MMS group was as follows: 17 (45%) patients with Stage I disease, 2 (5%) patients with Stage II disease, 19 (50%) patients with Stage III disease, and 0 (0%) patients with Stage IV disease, which was similar to that of the TVS group. Recently, a UK team reported on the final mortality, citing an overall average mortality reduction of 20%, and a reduction of 8% in years 0–7 and 28% in years 7–14 in the MMS group, compared with the no screening group [46]. They suggested that this late effect of screening was predictable given the unavoidable time interval from randomization to diagnosis and finally death. Therefore, their interpretation was that MMS screening was more effective after seven years of screening.

Very recently, Pavik pointed out two problems raised by the work of the UKCTOCS [53]. The UKCTOCS results from the analysis using the Cox proportional hazards model and the Royston–Parmar flexible parametric model indicated only small differences between the MMS and TVS modalities that were not statistically significant (estimated mortality reduction for years 7–14: 23% MMS vs. 21% TVS with the Royston–Parmar flexible parametric model). Another problem was that an expected lack of CA125 expression (20%) produces CA125-negative ovarian carcinomas that cannot be expected to be detected in the MMS group.

3.4. The Kentucky Screening Study

In the Kentucky Screening Study, single-arm annual TVS screenings of 37,293 women was performed [54,55]. The stage distribution of the 47 invasive ovarian cancers was as follows: 22 (47%) Stage I lesions, 11 (23%) Stage II lesions, 14 (30%) Stage III lesions, and 0 (0%) Stage IV lesions, with a 70% rate of Early-Stage (I/II) disease. The distribution of cancer histologies included 38% with serous carcinomas, 2% with mucinous carcinomas, 26% with endometrioid carcinomas, 4% with clear cell carcinomas, and 30% with others. The survival rate at five years of the patients with ovarian cancer in the annual screening group was better than that of the patients with ovarian cancer who did not undergo screening (74.8% ± 6.6% vs. 53.7% ± 2.3%, $p < 0.001$). Histologically, compared with the PLCO data, the rate of serous carcinomas was relatively low and the rate of endometrioid carcinomas was relatively high.

The authors concluded that annual TVS screening was associated with a decreased stage at detection, as well as a decrease in the case-specific ovarian cancer mortality. However, this study was not an RCT.

3.5. The Japanese Study

In Japan, the results of the Shizuoka Cohort Study of Ovarian Cancer Screening have been reported [56]. This study was an RCT of 82,487 low-risk postmenopausal women (intervention group: 41,688, control group: 40,799) who were screened using annual TVS and CA125 levels. The total number of cases of ovarian cancer in the screening group was 27 (0.06%). The stage distribution in the intervention group was as follows: 17 (63%) cases of Stage I disease, 1 (4%) case of Stage II disease, 7 (26%) cases of Stage III disease, and 2 (7%) cases of Stage IV disease. The distribution of the cancer histologies included 8 (30%) cases of serous carcinomas, 4 (15%) cases of mucinous carcinomas, 5 (19%) cases of endometrioid carcinomas, 9 (33%) cases of clear cell carcinomas, and 1 (4%) case of "other". Histologically, most of these cases involved cancers other than serous carcinoma. The proportion of Stage I/II ovarian cancers was higher in the screening group (67%) than in the control group (44%). The rate of complete surgical excision was higher in the screening group (21; 78%) than in the control group (15; 47%) ($p = 0.018$). However, the mortality rates are unknown, which again is problematic.

4. Differing Histological Subtypes of Ovarian Carcinoma among Races

In Europe, the USA, and Asia, there are significant differences in the rates of histological subtypes of ovarian carcinoma [57–62]. As we reported previously, the rate of aggressive ovarian cancer such as high-grade serous cancer (Type II) is significantly higher in Europe and the USA than in Asia ($p < 0.001$) [47]. For example, the rates of Type I vs. Type II are, 24% vs. 48% in Europe (including the UK); 24% vs. 66% in Denmark; and 30% vs. 45% in the USA. Conversely, Type I carcinomas—indolent carcinomas arising from precursors—are relatively common in Asia. For example, the rates of Type I vs. Type II are 53% vs. 33% in Japan; 58% vs. 24% in Hong Kong; and 66% vs. 34% in

Korea. These results theoretically imply that ovarian cancer screening using CA125/TVS would be more effective in Asia than in Europe and the USA, as the precursors or ovarian cancer can be detected at an earlier stage, thereby reducing the mortality.

5. Conclusions

We presented characteristics of subtypes of ovarian cancer, summarized in Table 1. Type I carcinomas are generally slow-growing indolent neoplasms, and their precursor lesions in the ovaries have clearly been described and are easily detected. Conversely, Type II carcinomas are clinically aggressive neoplasms and may develop de novo from the tubal and/or ovarian surface epithelium. The efficacy of ovarian cancer screening depends on the subtypes of ovarian cancer. Type I ovarian carcinomas are relatively common in Asia, while Type II ovarian carcinomas are relatively common in Europe and the USA. Therefore, annual ovarian cancer screening may improve the prognoses in Asia to a substantially greater degree than in Europe and the USA, as precursors or early-stage Type I ovarian carcinomas can be detected using CA125/TVS in those regions. Furthermore, it is possible to improve the prognosis or induce down-staging of Type II ovarian carcinomas, even in Europe and the USA. The detection of Type II ovarian carcinoma at an early stage remains an unresolved issue. We have likely failed to notice the presence of STICs using CA125/TVS screening alone, as neither method showed positive findings in women with STICs. Biomarkers for the early detection of Type II carcinomas such as STICs are therefore urgently needed [53].

Table 1. Characteristics of two types of ovarian carcinoma.

	Type I	Type II
Behavior	Indolent	Aggressive
Genetic instability	Not very unstable	Very unstable
TP 53 mutation	Low	High
BRCA1/BRCA2 mutation	Low	High
Ki 67 proliferative index	10%–15%	50%–75%
Histological subtype	Endometrioid Clear cell Mucinous Low grade serous	High grade serous
Precursor	Benign cyst	s/o Tubal dysplasia (de novo starting)
Discover a precursor	Easy	Difficult
Incidence	Asia > Europe, USA	Europe, USA > Asia

Acknowledgments: We would like to thank Christine D. Berg and PLCO Project Team who graciously sent the PLCO data to us. We also thank John Rensselaer van Nagell Jr. and Edward John Pavlik for offering the data of the Kentucky Screening Study.

Author Contributions: Masafumi Koshiyama wrote the paper. Noriomi Matsumura and Ikuo Konishi contributed to the design and preparation of the paper.

Conflicts of Interest: The authors declare no conflict of interest.

References

1. Ozor, R.F.; Rubin, S.C.; Thomas, G.M.; Robboy, S.J. Epithelial ovarian cancer. In *Principles and Practice of Gynecologic Oncology*; Hoskin, W.J., Perez, C.A., Young, R.C., Eds.; Lippincott Williams & Wilkins: Philadelphia, PA, USA, 2000; pp. 981–1057.
2. Buys, S.S.; Partridge, E.; Greene, M.H.; Prorok, P.C.; Reding, D.; Riley, T.L.; Hartge, P.; Fagerstrom, R.M.; Ragard, L.R.; Chia, D.; et al. Ovarian cancer screening in the Prostate, Lung, Colorectal and Ovarian (PLCO) Cancer Screening Trial: Findings from the initial screen of a randomized trial. *Am. J. Obstet. Gynecol.* **2005**, *193*, 1630–1639. [CrossRef] [PubMed]

3. Buys, S.S.; Patridge, E.; Black, A.; Johnson, C.C.; Lamerato, L.; Isaacs, C.; Reding, D.; Greenlee, R.T.; Yokochi, L.A.; Kessel, B.; et al. Effect of screening on ovarian cancer mortality: The Prostate, Lung, Colorectal and ovarian (PLCO) cancer screening randomized controlled trial. *JAMA* **2011**, *305*, 2295–2303. [CrossRef] [PubMed]
4. Koshiyama, M.; Matsumura, N.; Konishi, I. Recent concepts of ovarian carcinogenesis: Type I and Type II. *Biomed. Res. Int.* **2014**, *2014*, 934261. [CrossRef] [PubMed]
5. Horiuchi, A.; Itoh, K.; Shimizu, M.; Nakai, I.; Yamazaki, T.; Kimura, K.; Suzuki, A.; Shiozawa, I.; Ueda, N.; Konishi, I. Toward understanding the natural history of ovarian carcinoma development: A clinicopathological approach. *Gynecol. Oncol.* **2003**, *88*, 309–317. [CrossRef]
6. Van Gorp, T.; Amant, F.; Neven, P.V. Endometriosis and the development of malignant tumors of the pelvis. A review of literature. *Best Pract. Res. Clin. Obstet. Gynecol.* **2004**, *18*, 349–371. [CrossRef] [PubMed]
7. Mandai, M.; Yamaguchi, K.; Matsumura, N.; Konishi, I. Ovarian cancer in endometriosis:molecular biology, pathology, and clinical management. *Int. J. Clin. Oncol.* **2009**, *14*, 383–391. [CrossRef] [PubMed]
8. Mandai, M.; Matsumura, N.; Baba, T.; Yamaguchi, K.; Hamanishi, J.; Konishi, I. Ovarian clear cell carcinoma as a stress-responsive cancer: Influence of the microevirinment on the carcinogenesis and cancer phenotype. *Cancer Lett.* **2011**, *310*, 129–133. [CrossRef] [PubMed]
9. Yamaguchi, K.; Mandai, M.; Toyokuni, S.; Hamanishi, J.; Higuchi, T.; Takakura, K.; Fujii, S. Contents of endometriotic cysts, especially the high concentration of free iron, are a possible cause of carcinogenesis in the cysts through the iron-induced persistent oxidative stress. *Clin. Cancer Res.* **2008**, *4*, 32–40. [CrossRef] [PubMed]
10. Coquelle, A.; Toledo, F.; Stern, S.; Bieth, A.; Debatisse, M. A new role for hypoxia in tumor progression: Induction of fragile site triggering genomic rearrangements and formation of complex DMs and HSRs. *Mol. Cell* **1998**, *2*, 259–265. [CrossRef]
11. Meng, A.X.; Jalali, F.; Cuddihy, A.; Chan, N.; Bindra, R.S.; Glazer, P.M.; Bristow, R.G. Hypoxia down-regulates DNA double strand break repair gene expression in prostate cancer cells. *Radiother. Oncol.* **2005**, *76*, 168–176. [CrossRef] [PubMed]
12. Abou-Taleb, H.; Yamaguchi, K.; Matsumura, N.; Murakami, R.; Nakai, H.; Higasa, K.; Amano, Y.; Abiko, K.; Yoshioka, Y.; Hamanishi, J.; et al. Comprehensive assessment of the expression of the SWI/SNF complex defines two distinct prognosis subtypes of ovarian clear cell carcinoma. *Oncotarget* **2016**, *7*, 54758–54770. [PubMed]
13. Czriker, M.; Dockerty, M. Mucinous cystadenomas and mucinous cystadenocarcinomas of the ovary; a clinical and pathological study of 355 cases. *Cancer* **1954**, *7*, 302–310. [CrossRef]
14. Woodruff, J.D.; Bie, L.S.; Sherman, R.J. Mucinous tumors of the ovary. *Obstet. Gynecol.* **1960**, *16*, 699–712. [PubMed]
15. Rutgers, J.; Scully, R.E. Ovarian mullerian mucinous papillary cystadenomas of borderline malignancy. A clinicopathologic analysis. *Cancer* **1988**, *61*, 340–348. [CrossRef]
16. Lim, D.; Oliva, E. Precursors and pathogenesis of ovarian carcinoma. *Pathology* **2013**, *45*, 229–242. [CrossRef] [PubMed]
17. Mandai, M.; Konishi, I.; Kuroda, H.; Komatsu, T.; Yamamoto, S.; Nanbu, K.; Matsushita, K.; Fumumoto, M.; Yamabe, H.; Mori, T. Heterogeneous distribution of K-RAS-mutated epithelia in mucinous ovarian tumors with special reference to histopathology. *Hum. Pathol.* **1998**, *29*, 34–40. [CrossRef]
18. Enomoto, T.; Weghorst, C.M.; Inoue, M.; Tanizawa, O.; Rice, J.M. K-RAS activation occurs frequently in mucinous adenocarcinomas and rarely in other common epithelial tumors of the human ovary. *Am. J. Pathol.* **1991**, *139*, 777–785. [PubMed]
19. Ichikawa, Y.; Nishida, M.; Suzuki, H.; Yoshida, S.; Tsunoda, H.; Kudo, T.; Uchida, K.; Miwa, M. Mutation of KRAS protooncogene is associated with histological subtypes in human mucinous ovarian tumors. *Cancer Res.* **1994**, *54*, 33–35. [PubMed]
20. Caduff, R.F.; Svoboda-Newman, S.M.; Ferguson, A.W.; Johnston, C.M.; Frank, T.S. Comparison of mutations of Ki-RAS and p53 immmunoreactivity in borderline and malignant epithelial ovarian tumors. *Am. J. Surg. Pathol.* **1999**, *23*, 323–328. [CrossRef] [PubMed]
21. Gemignani, M.L.; Schlaerth, A.C.; Bogomolniy, F.; Barakat, R.R.; Lin, O.; Soslow, R.; Venkatraman, E.; Royd, J. Role of *KRAS* and *BRAF* gene mutations in mucinous ovarian carcinoma. *Gynecol. Oncol.* **2003**, *90*, 378–381. [CrossRef]

22. Mok, S.C.; Bell, D.A.; Knapp, R.C.; Fishbaugh, P.M.; Welch, W.R.; Muto, M.G.; Berkowitz, R.S.; Tsao, S.W. Mutation of K-RAS protooncogene in human ovarian epithelial tumors of borderline malignancy. *Cancer Res.* **1993**, *53*, 1489–1492. [PubMed]

23. Singer, G.; Stohr, R.; Cope, L.; Dehari, R.; Hartmann, A.; Cao, D.F.; Wang, T.L.; Kurman, R.J.; Shih, I.M. Patterns of p53 mutations separate ovarian serous borderline tumors and low- and high-grade carcinomas and provide support for a new model of ovarian carcinogenesis: A mutational analysis with immunohistochemical correlation. *Am. J. Surg. Pathol.* **2005**, *29*, 218–224. [CrossRef] [PubMed]

24. Pradham, M.; Davidson, B.; Trope, C.G.; Danielsen, H.E.; Abeler, V.M.; Risberq, B. Gross genomic alteration differ between serous borderline tumors and serous adenocarcinomas-an image cytometric DNA ploidy analysis of 307 cases with histogenetic implications. *Virchows Arch.* **2009**, *454*, 677–683. [CrossRef] [PubMed]

25. Kuo, K.T.; Guan, B.; Feng, Y.; Mao, T.L.; Jinawath, N.; Wang, Y.; Kurman, R.J.; Shih, I.M.; Wang, T.L. Analysis of DNA copy number alterations in ovarian serous tumors identifies new molecular genetic changes in low-grade and high-grade carcinomas. *Cancer Res.* **2009**, *69*, 4036–4042. [CrossRef] [PubMed]

26. Feeley, K.M.; Wells, M. Precursor lesions of ovarian epithelial malignancy. *Histopathology* **2001**, *38*, 87–95. [CrossRef] [PubMed]

27. Lauchlan, S.C. The secondary Mullerian system. *Obstet. Gynecol. Surv.* **1972**, *27*, 133–146. [CrossRef] [PubMed]

28. Dubeau, L. The cell of origin of ovarian epithelial tumours. *Lancet Oncol.* **2008**, *9*, 1191–1197. [CrossRef]

29. Kurman, R.J.; Vang, R.; Junge, J.; Hannibai, C.G.; Kjaer, S.K.; Shih, I.M. Papillary tubal hyperplasia: The putative precursor of ovarian atypical proliferative (borderline) serous tumors, noninvasive implants, and endosalpingiosis. *Am. J. Surg. Pathol.* **2011**, *35*, 1605–1614. [CrossRef] [PubMed]

30. Li, J.; Abushahin, N.; Pang, S.; Xiang, L.; Chambers, S.K.; Fadare, O.; Kong, B.; Zheng, W. Tubal origin of "ovarian" low-grade serous carcinoma. *Mod. Pathol.* **2011**, *24*, 1488–1499. [CrossRef] [PubMed]

31. Koshiyama, M.; Konishi, I.; Mandai, M.; Komatsu, T.; Yamamoto, S.; Nanbu, K.; Mori, T. Immunohistochemical analysis of p53 protein and 72kDa heat shock protein (HSP72) expression in ovarian carcinomas: Correlation with clinicopathology and sex steroid receptor status. *Virchows Arch.* **1995**, *425*, 603–609. [CrossRef] [PubMed]

32. Santin, A.D.; Zhan, F.; Bellone, S.; Palmieri, M.; Cane, S.; Bignotti, E.; Anfossi, S.; Gokden, M.; Dunn, D.; Romann, J.J.; et al. Gene expression profiles in primary ovarian serous papillary tumors and normal ovarian epithelium: Identification of candidate molecular markers for ovarian cancer diagnosis and therapy. *Int. J. Cancer* **2004**, *112*, 14–25. [CrossRef] [PubMed]

33. Salani, R.; Kurman, R.J.; Giuntoli, R., II; Gardner, G.; Bristow, R.; Wang, T.L.; Shih, I.M. Assessment of TP53 mutation using purified tissue samples of ovarian serous carcinomas reveals a higher mutation rate than previously reportedand does not correlate with drug resistance. *Int. J. Gynecol. Cancer* **2008**, *18*, 487–491. [CrossRef] [PubMed]

34. Cho, K.R.; Shih, I.M. Ovarian cancer. *Ann. Rev. Pathol.* **2009**, *4*, 287–313. [CrossRef] [PubMed]

35. Christie, M.; Oehler, M.K. Molecular pathology of epithelial ovarian cancer. *J. Br. Menopause Soc.* **2006**, *12*, 57–63. [CrossRef] [PubMed]

36. Cancer Genome Atlas Research Network. Integrated genomic analyses of ovarian carcinoma. *Nature* **2011**, *474*, 609–615.

37. Verhaak, R.G.; Tamayo, P.; Yang, J.Y.; Hubbard, D.; Zhang, H.; Creighton, C.J.; Fereday, S.; Lawrence, M.; Carter, S.L.; Mermel, C.H.; et al. Cancer Genome Atlas Research Network: Prognostically relevant gene signatures of high-grade serous ovarian carcinoma. *J. Clin. Investig.* **2013**, *123*, 517–525. [PubMed]

38. Murakami, R.; Matsumura, N.; Mandai, M.; Yoshihara, K.; Tanabe, H.; Nakai, H.; Yamanoi, K.; Abiko, K.; Yoshioka, Y.; Hamanishi, J.; et al. Establishment of a novel histopathological classification of high-grade serous ovarian carcinoma correlated with prognostically distinct gene expression subtypes. *Am. J. Pathol.* **2016**, *186*, 1103–1113. [CrossRef] [PubMed]

39. Horikawa, N.; Abiko, K.; Matsumura, N.; Hamanishi, J.; Baba, T.; Yamaguchi, K.; Yoshioka, Y.; Koshiyama, M.; Konishi, I. Expression of vascular endothelial growth factor in ovarian cancer inhibits tumor immunity through the accumulation of myeloid-derived suppressor cells. *Clin. Cancer Res.* **2017**, *23*, 587–599. [CrossRef] [PubMed]

40. Piek, J.M.; van Diest, P.J.; Zweemer, R.P.; Janse, J.W.; Poort-Keesom, R.J.; Menko, F.H.; Gille, J.J.; Jonqsma, A.P.; Pals, G.; Kenemans, P.; et al. Dysplastic changes in prophylactically removed fallopian tubes of women predisposed to developing ovarian cancer. *J. Pathol.* **2001**, *195*, 451–456. [CrossRef] [PubMed]

41. Chen, E.Y.; Mehra, K.; Mehrad, M.; Ning, G.; Miron, A.; Mutter, G.L.; Monte, N.; Quade, B.J.; McKeon, F.D.; Yassin, Y.; et al. Secretory cell outgrowth, PAX2 and serous carcinogenesis in the fallopian tube. *J. Pathol.* **2010**, *222*, 110–116. [CrossRef] [PubMed]

42. Gross, A.L.; Kurman, R.J.; Vang, R.; Shih, I.M.; Visvanathan, K. Precursor lesions of high-grade serous ovarian carcinoma: Morphological and molecular characteristics. *J. Oncol.* **2010**, *2010*, 126295. [CrossRef] [PubMed]

43. Carcangiu, M.L.; Radice, P.; Manoukian, S.; Spatti, G.; Gobbo, M.; Penstti, V.; Crucianelli, R.; Pasini, B. Atypical epithelial proliferation in Fallopian tubes in prophylactic salpingo-oophorectomy specimens from *BRCA1* and *BRCA2* germline mutation carriers. *Int. J. Gynecol. Pathol.* **2004**, *23*, 35–40. [CrossRef] [PubMed]

44. Seidman, J.D.; Yemelyanova, A.; Zaino, R.J.; Kurman, R.J. The fallopian tube-peritoneal junction: A potential site of carcinogenesis. *Int. J. Gynecol. Pathol.* **2011**, *30*, 4–11. [CrossRef] [PubMed]

45. Flesken-Nikitin, A.; Hwang, C.I.; Cheng, C.Y.; Michurina, T.V.; Enikolopov, G.; Nikitin, A.Y. Ovarian surface epithelium at the junction area contains a cancer-prone stem cell niche. *Nature* **2013**, *495*, 241–245. [CrossRef] [PubMed]

46. Jacobs, I.J.; Menon, U.; Ryan, A.; Gentry-maharai, A.; Burnell, M.; Kalsi, J.K.; Amso, N.N.; Apostolidou, S.; Benjamin, E.; Cruickshank, D.; et al. Ovarian cancer screening and mortality in the UK collaborative trial of ovarian cancer screening (UKCTOCS): A randomized controlled trial. *Lancet* **2016**, *387*, 945–956. [CrossRef]

47. Koshiyama, M.; Matsumura, M.; Konishi, I. Clinical efficacy of ovarian cancer screening. *J. Cancer* **2016**, *25*, 1311–1316. [CrossRef] [PubMed]

48. Menon, U.; Gentry-Maharaj, A.; Hallett, R.; Ryan, A.; Burnell, M.; Sharma, A.; Lewis, S.; Davies, S.; Philpott, S.; Lopes, A.; et al. Sensitivity and specificity of multimodal and ultrasound screening for ovarian cancer, and stage distribution of detected cancers: Results of the prevalence screen of the UK Collaborative Trial of Ovarian Cancer Screening (UKCTOCS). *Lancet Oncol.* **2009**, *10*, 327–340. [CrossRef]

49. Sharma, A.; Gentr-Maharaj, A.; Burnell, M.; Fourkala, E.O.; Campbell, S.; Amso, N.; Seif, M.W.; Ryan, A.; Parmar, M.; Jacobs, I.; et al. Assessing the malignant potential of ovarian inclusion cysts in postmenomausal women within the UK Collaborative Trial of Ovarian Cancer Screening (UKCTOCS): A prospective cohort study. *Gynecol. Oncol.* **2012**, *119*, 207–219.

50. Sharma, A.; Apostolidou, S.; Burnell, M.; Fourkala, E.O.; Campbell, S.; Amso, N.; Seif, M.W.; Ryan, A.; Parmar, M.; Jacobs, I.; et al. Risk of epithelial ovarian cancer in asymptomatic women with ultrasound-detected ovarian masses: A prospective cohort study within the UK collaborative trial of ovarian cancer screening (UKCTOCS). *Ultrasound Obstet. Gynecol.* **2012**, *40*, 338–344. [CrossRef] [PubMed]

51. Skates, S.J.; Xu, F.J.; Yu, Y.H.; Sjövall, K.; Einhorn, N.; Chang, Y.C.; Bast, R.C., Jr.; Knapp, R.C. Toward an optimal algorithm for ovarian cancer screening with longitudinal tumormarkers. *Cancer* **1995**, *76*, 2004–2010. [CrossRef]

52. Skates, S.J. Ovarian cancer screening: Develop of the risk of ovarian cancer algorithm (ROCA) and ROCA screening trials. *Int. J. Gynecol. Cancer* **2012**, *22*, S24–S26. [CrossRef] [PubMed]

53. Pavlik, E.D. Ovarian cancer screening effectiveness: A realization from the UK collaborative trial of ovarian cancer screening. *Womens Health* **2016**, *12*, 475–479. [CrossRef] [PubMed]

54. van Nagell, J.R., Jr.; DePriest, P.D.; Ueland, F.R.; DeSimone, C.P.; Cooper, A.L.; McDonald, J.M.; Pavlik, E.J.; Kryscio, R.J. Ovarian cancer screening with annual tranvaginal sonography: Findings of 25,000 women screened. *Cancer* **2007**, *109*, 1887–1896. [CrossRef] [PubMed]

55. van Nagell, J.R., Jr.; Miller, R.W.; DeSimone, C.P.; Ueland, F.R.; Podzielinski, I.; Goodrich, S.T.; Elder, J.W.; Huang, B.; Kryscio, R.J.; Pavlik, E.J. Long-term survival of women with epithelial ovarian cancer detected by ultrasonographic screening. *Obstet. Gynecol.* **2011**, *118*, 1212–1221. [CrossRef] [PubMed]

56. Kobayashi, H.; Yamada, Y.; Sato, T.; Sakata, M.; Kawaguchi, R.; Kanayama, S.; Shigetomi, H.; Haruta, S.; Tsuji, Y.; Ueda, S.; et al. A randomized study of screening for ovarian cancer: A multicenter study in Japan. *Int. J. Gynecol. Cancer* **2008**, *18*, 414–420. [CrossRef] [PubMed]

57. Sperling, C.; Noer, M.C.; Christensen, I.J.; Nielsen, M.L.; Lidegaard, Ø.; Høgdall, C. Comorbidity is an independent prognosis factor for the survival of ovarian cancer: A Danish register-based cohort study from a clinical database. *Gynecol. Oncol.* **2013**, *129*, 97–102. [CrossRef] [PubMed]

58. Gram, I.T.; Lukanova, A.; Brill, I.; Lund, E.; Overvad, K.; Tjønneland, A.; Clavel-Chabbert-Buffet, N.; Bamia, C.; Trichopoulou, A.; Zylis, D.; et al. Cigarette smoking and risk of histological subtypes of epithelial ovarian cancer in the EPIC cohort study. *Int. J. Cancer* **2012**, *130*, 2204–2210. [CrossRef] [PubMed]

59. Goodman, M.; Howe, H.L. Descriptive epidemiology of ovarian cancer in the United State, 1992–1997. *Cancer* **2003**, *97*, 2615–2630. [CrossRef] [PubMed]

60. Japan Society of Obstetrics and Gynecology. Statistics of gynecologic tumors in Japan. *Acta Obstet. Gynaecol. Jpn.* **2012**, *64*, 1029–1141.

61. Wong, K.H.; Mang, O.W.; Au, K.H.; Law, S.C. Incidence, mortality, and survival trends of ovarian cancer in Hong Kong, 1997 to 2006: A population-based study. *Hong Kong Med. J.* **2012**, *18*, 466–474. [PubMed]

62. Chung, H.H.; Hwang, S.Y.; Jung, K.W.; Won, Y.J.; Shin, H.R.; Kim, J.W.; Lee, H.P. Gynecologic Oncology Committee of Korean Society of Obstetrics and Gynecology. Ovarian cancer incidence and survival in Korea: 1993–2002. *Int. J. Gynecol. Cancer* **2007**, *17*, 595–600. [CrossRef] [PubMed]

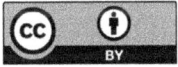

diagnostics

MDPI

Review

Psychological and Behavioral Impact of Participation in Ovarian Cancer Screening

Michael A. Andrykowski

Department of Behavioral Science, University of Kentucky College of Medicine, Lexington, KY 40536-0086, USA; mandry@uky.edu

Academic Editor: Andreas Kjaer
Received: 30 December 2016; Accepted: 6 March 2017; Published: 8 March 2017

Abstract: Evaluation of costs and benefits associated with cancer screening should include consideration of any psychological and behavioral impact associated with screening participation. Research examining the psychological and behavioral impact of screening asymptomatic women for ovarian cancer (OC) was considered. Research has focused upon potential negative psychological (e.g., distress) and behavioral (e.g., reduced future screening participation) impact of false positive (FP) OC test results. Results suggest FP OC screening results are associated with greater short-term OC-specific distress. While distress dissipates over time it may remain elevated relative to pre-screening levels for several weeks or months even after clinical follow-up has ruled out malignancy. The likelihood of participation in future OC screening may also be reduced. Research focused upon identification of any beneficial impact of participation in OC screening associated with receipt of "normal" results was also considered. This research suggests that a "normal" screening test result can have psychological benefits, including increased positive affect and beliefs in the efficacy of screening. It is concluded that any psychological or behavioral harms attributable to OC screening are generally very modest in severity and duration and might be counterbalanced by psychological benefits accruing to women who participate in routine OC screening and receive normal test results.

Keywords: ovarian cancer; psychological; psychosocial; behavioral; screening; false positive test result

1. Introduction

For some cancers, participation in cancer screening can lead to early diagnosis and an associated improvement in five-year survival. Consequently, great effort has been expended to develop cost-effective screening tests and protocols for cancers of the breast, colon, rectum, cervix, prostate, lung, and ovary—cancers with a high likelihood of treatment success when diagnosed and treated at an early stage of disease. Furthermore, for those screening tests for which the evidence suggests cost-effectiveness, great effort has been expended to ensure widespread uptake and appropriate repeat screening by screening-eligible individuals.

While participation in cancer screening can improve prognosis for some cancers, cancer screening is not without its drawbacks. All cancer screening approaches yield some proportion of inconclusive or abnormal results. These results typically require additional clinical follow-up to determine if a malignancy is present. Clinical follow-up might include surgery or biopsy, performance of a second-line screening test, or perhaps simply a repeat of the original screening test. In most instances, follow-up indicates the original abnormal or inconclusive screening test result is benign—no malignancy is present. Such false positive (FP) results may not be psychologically or behaviorally benign, however. A survey of recipients of FP test results in the context of breast, prostate, cervical or colorectal cancer screening found 40% described the experience as "very scary" or "the scariest time of my life" [1]. In general, research has shown a FP cancer screening test result can negatively impact both psychological (e.g., distress) and behavioral (e.g., participation in future cancer screening) outcomes [2–6], although research suggesting no impact is also available (e.g., [7]).

Recommendation of any cancer screening test for routine use in asymptomatic, average-risk women is based on the relative balance of the benefits and costs associated with that screening test. Identification of the benefits of any cancer screening test is relatively straightforward. Whether a cancer screening test results in a significant reduction in the number of deaths due to that specific cancer (i.e., cancer-specific mortality) is the primary determinant of the benefits of a particular screening test. A broader view of the benefits of a screening test could include consideration of any psychological or behavioral benefits associated with a screening test. Though rarely considered, participation in cancer screening may yield positive outcomes including reductions in cancer worry or increases in feelings of reassurance and well-being [8,9].

As one might expect, calculation of the costs of a screening test include consideration of the monetary costs associated with testing. In addition, calculation of the costs of a screening test should also include the "costs" associated with FP screening test results. These costs include the monetary as well as physical morbidity costs associated with performance of additional follow-up procedures or unnecessary surgeries. In addition, a FP screening test result might also exact certain psychological or behavioral costs. Psychological costs include fear or anxiety, a heightened sense of personal risk for cancer, or reduced confidence in the efficacy of the screening test, all of which might result in a significant behavioral cost—a lessened likelihood of returning for repeat screening in the future. If the collective costs associated with a screening test exceed the collective benefits of screening, one might well conclude that a particular screening test does more harm than good.

The purpose of this paper is to consider the literature regarding the psychological and behavioral impact of participation in routine screening for ovarian cancer (OC). Evidence regarding the potential for OC screening to yield both positive and negative psychological and behavioral outcomes will be considered.

2. Screening for Ovarian Cancer

When diagnosed and treated at a localized stage, OC is associated with a good prognosis. The five-year relative survival rate is 92% [10]. Unfortunately, the majority of cases of OC (61%) are diagnosed with late stage disease where existing treatment approaches are less likely to be successful and five-year relative survival rates are correspondingly only 27% [10]. Given this state of affairs, considerable effort has been expended to develop cost-effective approaches to screening for OC [11–16]. For the most part, these approaches include transvaginal ultrasonography (TVS) and serum tests for cancer antigen 125 (CA125), alone or in combination. While demonstrating some value in promoting early detection of OC in average-risk, asymptomatic women, no approach to OC screening has been shown to significantly reduce OC-specific mortality in asymptomatic, average-risk women in a prospective, randomized trial. As a result, implementation of routine screening for OC in asymptomatic, average-risk women has been controversial. Currently, the US Preventive Services Task Force recommends against routine screening for OC in asymptomatic, average-risk women (D recommendation) [17]. However, despite this recommendation, screening for OC is widely available and utilized for asymptomatic women at either average or elevated risk for OC. A recent survey of primary care physicians and obstetrician-gynecologists in the USA found many (33%) believed TVS and CA125 were effective screening tests for OC and many would offer OC screening tests to low (28%) and medium risk (65%) women [18].

3. Impact of False Positive OC Screening Test Results

Similar to screening tests for other cancers, screening for OC yields a certain proportion of inconclusive or abnormal test results [19]. For asymptomatic women at average risk for OC, approximately 5%–10% of OC screening tests yield an inconclusive or abnormal result, necessitating clinical follow-up. Fortunately, the vast majority of inconclusive or abnormal OC screening test results are ultimately deemed benign. While clinically benign, however, a FP OC screening test result may not be psychologically or behaviorally benign. An inconclusive or abnormal OC test result requiring additional clinical follow-up could understandably cause a woman to consider the possibility of a diagnosis of OC, resulting in a heightened sense of personal vulnerability. This in turn could result in the experience of fear, anxiety, and/or distress as well as a reduced likelihood of returning for future OC screening.

What is the evidence for such reactions? To answer this question a group of 10 studies are considered [20–29]. While an attempt was made to use PubMed to identify all relevant studies, a systematic review of the literature was not conducted and consequently no guarantee is made regarding the completeness of the studies considered here. Each of the 10 studies considered involves comparison of two groups of women participating in OC screening: women receiving a "normal" screening test result (i.e., Normal group) and women receiving an abnormal test result with clinical follow-up revealing no malignancy present (i.e., FP group). Comparison of these two groups of women has the potential to shed light on the impact of a FP OC screening test result. The specific OC screening test(s) employed varies across these studies but each employed CA125 testing or ultrasonography, typically transvaginal sonography (TVS), either alone or in combination. The psychological and behavioral outcomes the Normal and FP groups are compared upon vary widely across studies. The most common outcomes being generic mental health outcomes (e.g., state anxiety, depression, distress), OC-specific measures of distress and worry, OC risk perception, and participation in future cancer screening, either actual or stated intention to participate. These studies also vary widely with regard to study design (e.g., cross sectional vs. longitudinal), sample size in both the Normal and FP groups, and the timing of the assessment of outcomes (e.g., short-term vs long-term). Finally, some of these studies focused upon OC screening for women at intermediate or high risk for OC, typically due to a strong family history of OC [23,25–28]. The remaining studies focused upon OC screening among asymptomatic women generally at average risk for OC [20–22,24,29].

3.1. Impact of FP Results on Women at Intermediate or High Risk for OC

In an early study, 266 women at risk for familial OC underwent either transabdominal or transvaginal ultrasonagraphy with color Doppler imaging [27]. Women with abnormal results on initial scan returned in six weeks for a repeat scan. Women with repeat abnormal results at the repeat scan were referred for surgery. All women completed a questionnaire 6–15 weeks before the initial scan and again after their initial scan. Women also completed the same questionnaire after a repeat scan. Psychological outcomes assessed included OC risk perception, cancer worry, coping style, depression and anxiety symptoms, and general distress. Results indicated that following an initial scan, before a repeat scan ruled out the presence of malignancy, women receiving an abnormal result (*n* = 51) reported greater cancer worry, general distress, and anxiety than women receiving a normal scan result (i.e., Normal group; *n* = 189). Of women receiving an abnormal result at the initial scan, 32 received a normal result at the repeat scan and thus constituted a FP group. In the FP group, distress returned to baseline levels but remained elevated relative to the Normal group. Overall, it was concluded FP results are associated with increased distress in the short-term but this adverse impact is neither severe nor persistent.

Participants in this initial study completed the same study questionnaire as in the initial study one year after their initial scan [28]. In general, one year after their initial scan, women in the FP group did not differ from women in the Normal group with regard to distress and anxiety. However, more women in the FP group described themselves as "more worried" about cancer than women in the Normal group. It was concluded while FP results may be associated with some increased worry about cancer in the longer term, there is little evidence to suggest severe and persistent adverse psychological effects.

Kauff et al. examined women at intermediate risk for OC due to a personal or family history of breast and/or ovarian cancer but no documented BRCA1/2 mutation [25]. Women were offered semi-annual OC screening using TVS, CA125 testing, and pelvic examination. Women completed a baseline assessment at enrollment in the screening program and follow-up assessments every six months thereafter in conjunction with OC screening. Impact on mental quality of life (QOL) was indexed by the Mental Component Score of the Medical Outcome Study Short Form-36. At least one follow-up assessment was completed by 135 women. During a mean of 19.8 months of follow-up, 52 women experienced ≥1 abnormal OC screening test result. None of these women were ultimately deemed to have OC and constituted the FP group. Women in the FP group evidenced a clinically and statistically significant mean 6.4 point decrease in their Mental Component Score between baseline and their most recent follow-up assessment. (Lower scores represent poorer mental QOL). Women with no abnormal OC screening test result constituted the Normal group (n = 83) and evidenced a statistically and clinically insignificant mean 0.67 point drop in their Mental Component Score. It was concluded for women at intermediate risk for OC, FP screening results are associated with a significant decline in mental QOL.

As part of the United Kingdom Familial Ovarian Cancer Screening Study (OKFOCSS), women at increased genetic risk for OC (estimated lifetime risk >10%) participated in an OC screening program involving thrice yearly CA125 testing coupled with annual TVS [23]. If an abnormal test result occurred for either type of testing, women were recalled for retesting within two months. Women (n = 1999) completed a baseline assessment (T1) one month prior to an initial CA125 test and a follow-up assessment one week after receiving the result of this initial test (T2). Women receiving an abnormal test result at any time completed an additional follow-up one week after repeat of the screening test ruled out malignancy and they were returned to routine screening (T3). These women constituted the FP group (n = 167). The remaining women who received only normal test results during participation in the screening program constituted the Normal group. Finally, all women completed a final follow-up assessment nine months after receiving a normal test result (n = 825) or nine months after return to routine screening after receiving a FP result (n = 87) (T4). Specific outcomes assessed at each assessment included OC-specific distress, anxiety and depression symptoms, and reassurance. Compared to the Normal group the FP group reported moderately elevated OC-specific distress one week after being notified of their abnormal result. No difference in OC-specific distress was evident at T3 or T4, after women with FP results returned to routine screening. No differences with regard to anxiety, depression, or reassurance were noted between the Normal screening and FP groups at any assessment point. Finally, women in the FP group were significantly more likely to withdraw from the screening program (primarily for risk-reducing salpingo oophorectomy) (OR = 4.38). It was concluded FP screening results are associated with transient OC-specific distress but are not associated with sustained psychological harm.

Finally, 111 female BRCA1/2 mutation carriers who had not undergone risk-reducing surgery (i.e., salpingo oophorectomy) participated in a screening program involving both annual breast cancer screening and OC screening involving both CA125 testing and TVS [26]. All abnormal screening test results were followed by additional imaging and biopsy when appropriate. All participants completed a questionnaire prior to a baseline screening visit, as well as 3 and 12 months post-baseline. Psychological outcomes assessed included general anxiety, perceived absolute and comparative risk for OC, and OC worry. Women receiving normal OC screening test results following baseline screening constituted the Normal group and those receiving abnormal results with no cancer subsequently detected constituted a FP group. No significant differences were found between the Normal and FP groups for any of the OC risk or worry outcomes at either the 3 or 12 month follow-ups. Furthermore, there were no differences between the two groups in the likelihood of undergoing risk-reducing surgery. It was concluded FP test results were not associated with large increases in risk perception, cancer worry, or uptake of risk-reducing surgery. Unfortunately, only two women received abnormal CA125 test results (<2% of the sample) while the number of women receiving FP TVS test results was not reported. As a result, it is unclear whether the lack of significant findings might be due to a true absence of effect or simply due to inadequate statistical power.

3.2. Summary: Impact of FP Results on Women at Intermediate or High Risk for OC

Each of the studies considered in this group examined the impact of a FP screening test result on one or more psychological outcomes. Overall, the evidence suggests that a FP result in screening programs targeted at women at intermediate or high risk for OC is associated with significantly poorer psychological status in the immediate aftermath of an abnormal OC screening test result. This appears particularly true with regard to cancer-specific worry and distress [23,25,27]. Little evidence suggests much impact on more general indices of depression, anxiety or mental health or on perceptions of OC risk. Any impact on psychological status appears to be short-lived, however, as differences between FP and Normal groups generally decline over time following determination no malignancy is present [23,28]. The study by Kauff et al. [25] appears to be an exception to this general conclusion, however, as they found FP results were associated with significant and long-term declines in a generic measure of mental health. However, their data analytic strategy did not account for when a FP result was experienced in the course of the mean nearly 20 months of observation. This makes it difficult to attribute any observed declines in mental health status to the experience of a FP screening test result. Finally, Brain et al. found women receiving FP results were over four times more likely to withdraw from their OC screening program [23]. Withdrawal was typically followed by risk-reducing surgery, however, eliminating the need for further OC screening. It was unclear, however, whether women in the FP group were more likely than women in the Normal group to discontinue participation in OC screening in the absence of risk-reducing surgery. This is a critical missing piece of information given any risk-reducing impact of a screening program is predicated upon continued, appropriate participation with the program [30].

3.3. Impact of FP Results on Women at Average Risk for OC

The studies considered here examined the psychological and behavioral impact of a FP OC screening test result on asymptomatic women generally at average risk for OC [20–22,24,29]. Andersen et al. examined women (n = 592) at "conventional" risk for OC (i.e., ≤1 first degree relative with OC) undergoing alternating CA125 and TVS testing every six months for 18 months [20]. Abnormal CA125 results were followed by TVS screening while abnormal TVS results required repeat TVS screening in six to eight weeks. Measures of QOL, worry about OC risk, and OC-specific distress were completed at a baseline assessment prior to the initial OC screening test and a follow-up two years post-baseline, after the screening program was concluded. At follow-up, women receiving a FP OC screening test result at some point during the two-year screening period (n = 32) were compared to similar women who received normal screening test results (i.e., Normal group). The FP group reported significantly greater worry about OC risk. Cancer-specific distress and quality of life did not differ between the FP and Normal screening groups. It was concluded FP screening test results may have long-term effects and increase worry about cancer risk.

Barrett et al. examined the psychological impact of a FP screening test in women participating in the United Kingdom Collaborative Trial of Ovarian Cancer Screening (UKCTOCS), a randomized trial of annual multimodal OC screening [21]. Women (n = 202,638) were randomized to one of three arms: (1) OC screening with CA125 testing followed, if necessary, by TVS (CA125+TVS) as a second line test; (2) OC screening with TVS; or (3) no OC screening. Following receipt of an abnormal screening test result women in the CA125+TVS arm underwent a repeat CA125 test with (Level 2) or without (Level 1) TVS testing. Women in the TVS group underwent a repeat TVS test by a senior ultrasonographer within three months (Level 1) or a repeat TVS test or biopsy within six weeks (Level 2). All women completed a baseline questionnaire prior to randomization. Women in the two screening groups who received an abnormal screening test result (n = 22,035) completed a questionnaire following each abnormal screen and annually thereafter. The questionnaire included measures of state anxiety as well as general psychological morbidity as assessed by the General Health Questionnaire (GHQ-12). Results indicated greater psychological morbidity in women after receipt of a FP test result but only for women receiving more intensive repeat screening (i.e., Level 2 repeat screening). In other words, women in the CA125+TVS screening group exhibited greater psychological morbidity only if repeat screening involved repeat of both the CA125 and TVS tests while women in the TVS screening group exhibited greater psychological morbidity only if repeat screening involved a TVS scan or biopsy (i.e., Level 2 repeat screening). No differences between the FP and Normal groups were found for state anxiety. It was concluded a FP test results in slightly increased psychological morbidity when an abnormal screening test result is followed by more intensive forms of repeat screening.

The remaining studies in this group examined asymptomatic, average-risk women participating in an ongoing trial of OC screening using annual TVS at the University of Kentucky [22,24,29]. In this trial, an abnormal TVS test result requires repeat of the TVS screening test in 2–16 weeks. In an initial study [22], women (n = 540) completed a baseline assessment immediately before undergoing a routine annual TVS screening test and follow-up assessments two weeks and four months post-baseline. A single-item measure of OC risk perception (i.e., perceived lifetime personal risk) as well as measures of general and OC-specific distress were completed at all assessments. Women receiving a FP screening test result (n = 33) at baseline were compared to women receiving a normal screening test result (i.e., Normal group; n = 507). Compared to women receiving a "normal" TVS test result, women receiving a FP result reported significantly elevated OC-specific distress at the two-week follow-up, before a repeat TVS test had clarified whether a malignancy was present. Distress returned to baseline levels at four-month follow-up, after repeat of the TVS test indicated no malignancy was present. No differences between the FP and Normal groups on mood disturbance, depression, or OC risk perception were found. It was concluded a FP test result is associated with a significant, but transient, increase in OC-specific distress.

As a follow-up to this initial study, a larger longitudinal study examining psychological and behavioral responses to receipt of a FP OC screening test result was implemented [29]. Women receiving a FP TVS test result (n = 375) in the course of routine, annual TVS screening were compared to women (n = 375) receiving a normal test result (i.e., Normal group). Women in the FP group were matched with women in the Normal group with regard to age, family history of OC, and OC screening history (prior FP result, number of prior TVS tests). Women in the FP group completed a baseline assessment immediately prior to undergoing a repeat TVS test, required to clarify the nature of a recent abnormal TVS test 2 to 16 weeks earlier. Women in the Normal group completed a baseline assessment immediately prior to a routine, annual TVS screening test. Both groups completed follow-up assessments one and four months after baseline. Results indicated FP test results were associated with clinically significant increases in OC-specific distress with distress remaining elevated through the four month follow-up. Women receiving a FP result also reported significantly higher perceptions of OC risk on two different, two-item composite measures of risk (Personal OC Risk and Comparative OC Risk) and fewer perceived positive consequences of screening participation. A FP test result also impacted screening intentions as the FP group reported at one month follow-up significantly weaker intentions to return for future OC screening. No differences between the FP and Normal groups were found with regard to depressive symptoms, benefit finding, or beliefs in the effectiveness of OC screening at any of the study assessments. It was concluded FP results negatively impact both affective (OC-specific distress) and cognitive (risk perception) outcomes in both the short and intermediate term. The negative psychological impact of a FP test is still evident for several months after repeat testing has ruled out malignancy and may serve to reduce motivation to participate in future routine OC screening.

Finally, Floyd et al. examined the impact of a FP test result on women's interest in receiving health-related information [24]. Based on the possibility a FP screening test result could be experienced as a very scary and threatening event [1], it was hypothesized a FP result may serve as a "teachable moment" [31] and enhance interest in obtaining additional information about OC as well as other health-related topics. A Normal screening group (n = 124) consisted of women undergoing a routine, annual TVS test with receipt of normal results. This group completed a baseline assessment prior to undergoing routine TVS screening. A FP screening group (n = 279) consisted of women who had received an abnormal TVS test result 2–16 weeks earlier and were returning for a repeat TVS test to clarify whether a malignancy was present. These women completed a baseline assessment prior to undergoing this repeat TVS screening test. All women completed a follow-up assessment one month post-baseline where interest in receiving information about 10 different health- and cancer-related topics was assessed. Contrary to hypothesis, results indicated women receiving FP screening test results were significantly less interested in receiving health- and cancer-related information than women receiving normal screening results. It was concluded receipt of a FP result does not represent a teachable moment when women may be more receptive to health information and health behavior change. Rather receipt of a FP screening test result appears to make women less interested in health-related information, including information regarding OC.

3.4. Summary: Impact of FP Results on Women at Average Risk for OC

Most studies in this group examined the impact of a FP screening test result on one or more psychological outcomes [20–22,29]. In each of these studies, a negative impact on psychological outcomes was observed. Receipt of a FP result was associated with poorer psychological status, particularly OC-specific worry [20] and OC-specific distress [22,29]. Little evidence suggests FP results exert a significant impact on more general measures of psychological morbidity or distress, although one study did find elevated psychological morbidity in women receiving a FP result requiring more intense, invasive repeat testing after an abnormal result [21]. While it is clear FP results impact OC-specific distress, the duration of this impact is not completely clear. It is quite apparent receipt of an abnormal screening test result is associated with an immediate and pronounced spike in OC-specific distress [22,29] which remains elevated for at least several weeks or months even after repeat OC screening rules out malignancy [29]. Overall, the evidence suggests that receipt of a FP screening test result increases OC-specific distress and worry in the short term and quite possibly in the intermediate term. As for other outcomes, the data are sparse or mixed. The two studies that examined the impact of a FP test result on perceptions of OC risk yielded mixed results [22,29]. While one study found no impact upon OC risk perception [22], a larger and better designed study found a FP result resulted in higher perceptions of OC risk up to four months after repeat TVS testing ruled out malignancy [29]. The failure to find a significant impact on OC risk perception in the earlier study [22] could be due to a lack of statistical power as well as use of a relatively crude measure of OC risk perception. The earlier study [22] included only 33 women in the FP result group compared to 375 women in the later study [29], making it less likely a "true" impact on OC risk perception could be detected in the earlier study. Additionally, the earlier study indexed OC risk perception using only a single, single-item measure of risk perception. In contrast, the later study [29] found significant effects on two separate, two-item composite measures of OC risk perception. Finally, a FP result may impact the likelihood of participation in future screening as receipt of a FP result was associated with significantly weaker intentions to return for future OC screening [29].

4. Impact of Normal OC Screening Test Results

As might be expected, an abnormal or FP test result appears to have at least some negative impact on psychological and behavioral outcomes. Might the opposite be true? Does receipt of a "normal" OC screening test result yield a positive impact on psychological or behavioral outcomes? In contrast to the attention focused upon the impact of abnormal or FP results, it appears the impact of a "normal" test result on psychological and behavioral outcomes has received less attention. In an initial study, high-risk women (n = 275) underwent ultrasound screening for OC [32]. Nearly $\frac{3}{4}$ reported feeling reassured after screening. In a more recent and comprehensive study, asymptomatic, average-risk women (n = 560) completed a baseline assessment immediately prior to undergoing routine, annual TVS screening for OC as well as follow-up assessment two weeks and four months post-baseline [33]. All women received a "normal" screening test result. Growth curve modeling revealed receipt of a "normal" test result was associated with a significant decrease in OC-specific distress and significant increases in positive affect, belief in the efficacy of OC screening, and knowledge of OC risk factors between the baseline and four-month follow-up assessment. No effect was observed on OC risk perceptions, negative affect, or more generic measures of distress (i.e., depression, mood disturbance). It was concluded participation in routine OC screening with receipt of a normal result can positively impact affective and cognitive psychological outcomes that can serve to promote continued participation in OC screening.

5. Summary and Recommendations

Determination of the value of any cancer screening test requires careful consideration of the costs and benefits associated with that screening test. Obviously, certain types of costs and benefits are weighed more heavily than others. The paramount benefit of a screening test is the extent to which it reduces cancer-related mortality. On the cost side of the ledger, the economic and physical morbidity costs (e.g., surgeries) associated with a screening test are weighed most heavily. Less frequently considered are any psychological and behavioral costs and benefits associated with a cancer screening test.

The purpose of this paper was to consider the psychological and behavioral impact, both costs and benefits, associated with participation in OC screening. The studies we considered are diverse in methodology and design. Most of these studies focused upon documenting the psychological "costs" associated with abnormal, ultimately FP, OC screening test results. In general, these studies clearly suggest that women who experience a FP OC screening test result report more OC-specific worry and distress in the short-term [22,23,27,29]. This is unsurprising, of course, given receipt of an abnormal result raises at least the possibility of a subsequent diagnosis of OC. This distress appears to dissipate over time, but may still be present to a degree four months to a year or more after receipt of an abnormal result and after clinical follow-up has ruled out a malignancy [20,28,29]. This general conclusion appears to be true regardless of the OC risk status of the asymptomatic women being screened.

In contrast to the findings for OC-specific distress and worry, the impact of a FP screening test result on other psychological outcomes is less clear. The impact on generic measures of mental health, depression and anxiety is mixed with some research showing a negative impact [21,25,27] and other research showing no impact [20,22,23,29]. Similarly, the impact of a FP result on perceptions of OC risk is also mixed with some studies finding no impact [22,27] but another, larger, better-designed study finding increased perceptions of OC risk in women experiencing a FP result [29].

With regard to behavioral costs associated with a FP OC screening test result, FP test results may be associated with reduced future participation in OC screening [23] or reduced intentions to return for routine screening in the future [29]. Given the effectiveness of any cancer screening modality is predicated upon continued screening uptake at appropriate intervals, this is a significant potential cost associated with FP results in the OC screening setting.

In contrast to the negative impact of a FF OC screening test result, it appears woman may benefit from participation in routine OC screening when a "normal" screening test result is received. For asymptomatic, average-risk women, participation in OC screening with receipt of a "normal" test result was associated with a significant decrease in OC-specific distress and significant increases in positive affect, belief in the efficacy of OC screening, and knowledge of OC risk factors over a four month period following screening [33]. Additionally, comparison of women receiving FP and normal results found women receiving normal screening test results attributed more positive consequences to their screening experience such as greater feelings of well-being and reassurance [29]. This data is provocative in its suggestion that participation in screening may not be a completely benign experience from a psychological and behavioral standpoint. Rather, participation in screening may create affective and cognitive conditions that may not only be inherently positive and reinforcing, but may also serve to further promote continued participation in OC screening.

While showing some ability to detect OC at an earlier stage, randomized trials have failed to show a reduction in cancer-specific mortality in asymptomatic, average-risk women participating in OC screening programs. Coupled with consideration of the monetary costs of OC screening and the potential physical morbidity costs (e.g., surgery) associated with FP test results, the US Preventive Services Task Force recommends against routine screening for OC in asymptomatic, average-risk women (D recommendation) [17]. Despite this negative recommendation, routine screening of asymptomatic women at average risk for OC is unlikely to go away. OC screening is well accepted by many physicians [18] as well as by the public. An overwhelming majority of women participating in the University of Kentucky OC screening program indicated they agreed or strongly agreed that TVS screening is effective in the early diagnosis of OC [29]. As a result, further research on the psychological and behavioral impact of participation in OC screening is warranted. While more research is needed, what is particularly needed is better research. Future research examining the impact of FP screening test results should be characterized by (1) sufficient numbers of women receiving abnormal or FP results to ensure adequate statistical power and the ability to interpret null findings; (2) longitudinal assessment to enable identification of the duration of impact of a specific abnormal or FP test result on key psychological and behavioral outcomes; and (3) removal of women who undergo risk-reducing oophorectomy from analyses focused upon understanding the impact of FP results on future screening participation.

In addition, there is likely benefit from expanding the focus of research regarding the psychological and behavioral impact of participation in OC screening. In particular, more research is needed regarding the potential impact of participation in routine OC screening with receipt of a "normal" test result. While research has examined the potential positive impact of a normal test result [33] the potential negative impact of a normal test result has received scant, if any, attention. Potential negative impact might involve delay in help-seeking following any subsequent onset of symptoms related to OC or a general complacency about health. Two other areas are also largely unexamined: the psychological and behavioral impact of false negative OC screening test results—receipt of a normal screening test result when OC is present—and the impact of true positive OC screening test results. In the latter case, the psychological and behavioral impact of a diagnosis of OC may differ depending on whether OC was screening- or symptomatically-detected.

In conclusion, the research considered here does not suggest that FP test results in the course of screening asymptomatic women for OC result in significant, durable psychological harm. In addition, there is some suggestion that participation in routine screening for OC may confer psychological benefits. Some have contended OC screening "does more harm than good" [34]. If true, this contention is true based largely on consideration of the physical harms associated with surgeries performed for diagnostic or preventive purposes following abnormal OC screening results. Any psychological or behavioral harms attributable to OC screening appear to be, at worst, rather modest in severity and duration and might well be counterbalanced by psychological benefits accruing to women who participate in routine OC screening and who receive normal test results.

Conflicts of Interest: The author declare no conflict of interest.

References

1. Schwartz, L.M.; Woloshin, S.; Fowler, F.J., Jr.; Welch, H.G. Enthusiasm for cancer screening in the United States. *J. Am. Med. Assoc.* **2004**, *291*, 71–78. [CrossRef] [PubMed]
2. Brewer, N.T.; Salz, T.; Lillie, S.E. Systematic review: The long-term effects of false-positive mammograms. *Ann. Intern. Med.* **2007**, *146*, 502–510. [CrossRef] [PubMed]
3. Lin, K.; Lipsitz, R.; Miller, T.; Janakiraman, S. Benefits and harms of prostate-specific antigen screening for prostate cancer: An evidence update for the U.S. Preventive services task force. *Ann. Intern. Med.* **2008**, *149*, 192–199. [CrossRef] [PubMed]

4. Slatore, C.G.; Sullivan, D.R.; Pappas, M.; Humphrey, L.L. Patient-centered outcomes among lung cancer screening recipients with computed tomography: A systematic review. *J. Thorac. Oncol.* **2014**, *9*, 927–934. [CrossRef] [PubMed]

5. Taylor, K.L.; Shleby, R.; Gelmann, E.; McGuire, C. Quality of life and trial adherence among participants in the prostate, lung, colorectal, and ovarian cancer screening trial. *J. Natl. Cancer Inst.* **2004**, *96*, 1083–1094. [CrossRef] [PubMed]

6. Wardle, J.; Pope, R. The psychological costs of screening for cancer. *J. Psychosom. Res.* **1992**, *36*, 609–624. [CrossRef]

7. O'Sullivan, I.; Sutton, S.; Dixon, S.; Perry, N. False positive results do not have a negative effect on reattendance for subsequent breast screening. *J. Med. Screen* **2001**, *8*, 145–148. [CrossRef] [PubMed]

8. Cockburn, J.; de Luise, T.; Hurley, S.; Clover, K. Development and validation of the PCQ: A questionnaire to measure the psychological consequences of screening mammography. *Soc. Sci. Med.* **1992**, *34*, 1129–1134. [CrossRef]

9. Tyndel, S.; Austoker, J.; Henderson, B.J.; Brain, K.; Bankhead, C.; Clements, A.; Watson, E.K. What is the psychological impact of mammographic screening on younger women with a family history of breast cancer? Findings from a prospective cohort study by the PIMMS Management Group. *J. Clin. Oncol.* **2007**, *25*, 3823–3830. [CrossRef] [PubMed]

10. *Cancer Facts and Figures*; American Cancer Society: Atlanta, GA, USA, 2015.

11. Buys, S.S.; Partridge, E.; Black, A.; Johnson, C.C.; Lamerato, L.; Isaacs, C.; Reding, D.J.; Greenlee, R.T.; Yokochi, L.A.; Kessel, B.; et al. Effect of screnning on ovarian cancer mortality: The Prostate, Lung, and Ovarian (PLCO) Cancer Screening randomized controlled trial. *J. Am. Med. Assoc.* **2011**, *305*, 2295–2303. [CrossRef] [PubMed]

12. Jacobs, I.J.; Menon, U.; Ryan, A.; Gentry-Maharaj, A.; Burnell, M.; Kalsi, J.K.; Amso, N.N.; Apostolidou, E.B.; Cruickshank, D.; Crump, D.N.; et al. Ovarian cancer screening and mortality in the UK Collaborative Trial of Ovarian Cancer Screening (UKCTOS): A randomised controlled trial. *Lancet* **2016**, *387*, 945–956. [CrossRef]

13. Menon, U.; Griffin, M.; Gentry-Maharaj, A. Ovarian cancer screening—Current status, future directions. *Gynecol. Oncol.* **2014**, *132*, 490–495. [CrossRef] [PubMed]

14. Reade, C.J.; Riva, J.J.; Busse, J.W.; Goldsmith, C.H.; Elit, L. Risks and benefits of screening asymptomatic women for ovarian cancer: A systematic review and meta-analysis. *Gynecol. Oncol.* **2013**, *130*, 674–681. [CrossRef] [PubMed]

15. Schorge, J.O.; Modesitt, S.C.; Coleman, R.L.; Cohn, D.E.; Kauff, N.D.; Duska, L.R.; Herzog, T.J. SGO white paper on ovarian cancer: Etiology, screening and surveillance. *Gynecol. Oncol.* **2010**, *119*, 7–17. [CrossRef] [PubMed]

16. Van Nagell, J.R., Jr.; Pavlik, E.J. Ovarian cancer screening. *Clin. Obstet. Gynecol.* **2012**, *55*, 43–51. [CrossRef] [PubMed]

17. Moyer, V.A. U.S. Preventive Services Task Force. Screening for ovarian cancer: U.S. Preventive Services Task Force reaffirmation recommendation statement. *Ann. Intern. Med.* **2012**, *157*, 900–904. [CrossRef] [PubMed]

18. Baldwin, L.-M.; Trivers, K.F.; Matthews, B.; Andrilla, C.H.A.; Miller, J.W.; Berry, D.L.; Lishner, D.M.; Goff, B.A. Vignette-based study of ovarian cancer screening: Do U.S. physicians report adhering to evidence-based recommendations. *Ann. Intern. Med.* **2012**, *156*, 182–194. [CrossRef] [PubMed]

19. Pavlik, E.J.; Ueland, F.R.; Miller, R.V.V.; Ubellacker, J.M.; DeSimone, C.P.; Hoff, J.; Baldwin, R.J.; Kryscio, R.J.; van Nagell, J.R., Jr. Frequency and disposition of ovarian abnormalities followed with serial transvaginal sonography. *Obstet. Gynecol.* **2013**, *122*, 210–217. [CrossRef] [PubMed]

20. Andersen, M.R.; Drescher, C.W.; Zheng, Y.; Bowen, D.J.; Wilson, S.; Young, A.; McIntosh, M.; Mahony, B.S.; Lowe, K.A.; Urban, N. Changes in cancer worry associated with participation in ovarian cancer screening. *Psychooncology* **2007**, *16*, 814–820. [CrossRef] [PubMed]

21. Barrett, J.; Jenkins, V.; Farewell, V.; Menon, U.; Jacobs, I.; Kilkerr, J.; Ryan, A.; Langridge, C.; Fallowfield, L.; UKCTOCS Trialists. Psychological morbidity associated with ovarian cancer screening: Results from more than 23,000 women in the randomised trial of ovarian cancer screening (UKCTOCS). *BJOG* **2014**, *121*, 1071–1079. [CrossRef] [PubMed]

22. Andrykowski, M.A.; Boerner, L.M.; Salsman, J.M.; Pavlik, E. Psychological response to test results in an ovarian cancer screening program: A prospective, longitudinal study. *Health Psychol.* **2004**, *23*, 622–630. [CrossRef] [PubMed]

23. Brain, K.E.; Lifford, K.J.; Fraser, L.; Rosenthal, A.N.; Rogers, M.T.; Lancastle, D.; Phelps, C.; Watson, E.K.; Clements, A.; Menon, U. Psychological outcomes of familial ovarian cancer screening: No evidence of long-term harm. *Gynecol. Oncol.* **2012**, *127*, 556–563. [CrossRef] [PubMed]

24. Floyd, A.; Steffens, R.F.; Pavlik, E.; Andrykowski, M.A. Receipt of a false positive test result during routine screening for ovarian cancer: A teachable moment? *J. Clin. Psychol. Med. Settings* **2011**, *18*, 70–77. [CrossRef] [PubMed]

25. Kauff, N.D.; Hurley, K.E.; Hensley, M.L.; Robson, M.E.; Lev, G.; Goldfrank, D.; Castiel, M.; Brown, C.L.; Ostroff, J.S.; Hann, L.E.; et al. Ovarian carcinoma screening in women at intermediate risk: Impact on quality of life and need for invasive follow-up. *Cancer* **2005**, *104*, 314–320. [CrossRef] [PubMed]

26. Portnoy, D.B.; Loud, J.T.; Han, P.K.J.; Mai, P.L.; Greene, M.H. Effects of false-positive cancer screenings and cancer worry on risk-reducing surgery among BRCA1/2 carriers. *Health Psychol.* **2015**, *34*, 709–717. [CrossRef] [PubMed]

27. Wardle, J.; Collins, W.; Pernet, A.L.; Whitehead, M.I.; Bourne, T.H.; Campbell, S. Psychological impact of screening for familial ovarian cancer. *J. Natl. Cancer Inst.* **1993**, *85*, 653–657. [CrossRef] [PubMed]

28. Wardle, J.; Pernet, A.; Collins, W.; Bourne, T. False positive results in ovarian cancer screening: One year follow-up of psychological status. *Psychol. Health* **1994**, *10*, 33–40. [CrossRef]

29. Wiggins, A.; Pavlik, E.J.; Andrykowski, M.A. Affective, cognitive, and behavioral outcomes associated with a false positive screening test for ovarian cancer. *J. Behav. Med.* **2017**, in press.

30. Weller, D.P.; Campbell, C. Uptake in cancer screening programmes: A priority in cancer control. *Br. J. Cancer* **2009**, *101* (Suppl. 2), S55–S59. [CrossRef] [PubMed]

31. McBride, C.M.; Emmons, K.M.; Lipkus, I.M. Understanding the potential of teachable moments: The case of smoking cessation. *Health Educ. Res.* **2003**, *18*, 156–170. [CrossRef] [PubMed]

32. Andolf, E.; Jorgensen, C.; Uddenberg, N.; Ursing, I. Psychological effects of ultrasound screening for ovarian carcinoma. *J. Psychosom. Obstet. Gynaecol.* **1990**, *11*, 155–162. [CrossRef]

33. Gaugler, J.E.; Pavlik, E.; Salsman, J.M.; Andrykowski, M.A. Psychological and behavioral impact of receipt of a "normal" ovarian cancer screening test. *Prev. Med.* **2006**, *42*, 463–470. [CrossRef] [PubMed]

34. Slomski, A. Screening women for ovarian cancer still does more harm than good. *J. Am. Med. Assoc.* **2012**, *307*, 2474–2475. [CrossRef] [PubMed]

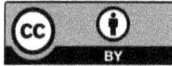

diagnostics

MDPI

Opinion

A Perspective on Ovarian Cancer Biomarkers: Past, Present and Yet-To-Come

Frederick R. Ueland

Department of Obstetrics and Gynecology, Division of Gynecologic Oncology and the Markey Cancer Center, University of Kentucky College of Medicine, Lexington, KY 40515, USA; fuela0@uky.edu; Tel.: +1-859-257-1613

Academic Editor: Andreas Kjaer
Received: 7 January 2017; Accepted: 23 February 2017; Published: 8 March 2017

Abstract: The history of biomarkers and ultrasonography dates back over more than 50 years. The present status of biomarkers used in the context of ovarian cancer is addressed. Attention is given to new interpretations of the etiology of ovarian cancer. Cancer antigen 125 (CA125) and multivariate index assays (Ova1, Risk of Ovarian Malignancy Algorithm, Overa) are biomarker-driven considerations that are presented. Integration of biomarkers into ovarian cancer diagnostics and screening are presented in conjunction with ultrasound. Consideration is given to the serial application of both biomarkers and ultrasound, as well as morphology-based indices. Attempts are made to foresee how individualized molecular signatures may be able to both provide an alert of the potential for ovarian cancer and to provide molecular treatments tailored to a personalized genetic signature. In the future, an annual pelvic ultrasound and a comprehensive serum biomarker screening/diagnostic panel may replace the much maligned bimanual examination as part of the annual gynecologic examination. Taken together, it is likely that a new medical specialty for screening and early diagnostics will emerge for physicians and epidemiologists, a field of study that is independent of patient gender, organ, or the subspecialties of today.

Perspective

Ghost of Christmas Yet-To-Come

Original illustration by John Leech, 1843

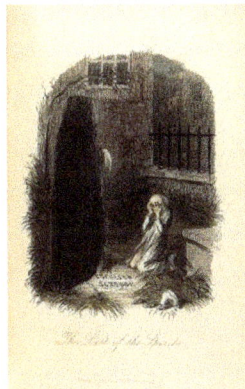

Keywords: biomarkers; ovarian tumor biomarkers; ultrasound; serial ultrasound; ovarian cancer

As one year closes and another begins, I find myself reflecting on ovarian cancer diagnostics. It is truly humbling how little we have accomplished in this field over the last half-century. All the while, the rest of the world has been busy. Since the first biomarker was reported, we have harnessed the atom and ushered in the Nuclear Age. Since the first *ovarian* biomarker was reported, we have invented the integrated circuit and spawned the dynamic Information Age. Yet, as gynecologic oncologists, we continue to struggle with the early identification of ovarian cancer and whether ovarian cancer actually begins in the ovary at all. The first serum biomarker for epithelial ovarian cancer was introduced in 1965 (carcinoembyonic antigen, CEA) [1]. This was a milestone in cancer diagnostics, as prior to this, oncologists were equipped with little to detect or monitor ovarian cancer. Keep in mind that this was when ultrasound was just emerging as a very rudimentary medical diagnostic instrument, and well before the advent of computed tomography (CT) or magnetic resonance imaging (MRI). Now some fifty years later, it is easy to ask, "Why haven't we done more?" Perhaps the recent focus on molecular-genetic technology and personalized cancer treatment will inspire a new Diagnostic Age in oncology. I am an optimist at heart, and am hopeful that our biomarker story will read somewhat like the Charles Dickens novella, A Christmas Carol, where the return of Jacob Marley's ghost 7 years after his death helps give clarity to the past, present, and yet-to-come.

First, it is important to clarify our diagnostic objective. My generation has believed, quite sensibly I think, that epithelial ovarian cancer arises from the ovary. Ovarian cancer has always utilized a taxonomy-based classification system first introduced in the 1930s, then validated by the World Health Organization's Classification in 1973, and propagated into modern day. The story was as follows: ovarian epithelial inclusion cysts are trapped beneath the surface epithelium of the ovary and eventually undergo malignant transformation giving rise to invasive cancer. It was all a little mysterious and the association with ovulation was difficult to validate, but "incessant ovulation" did appear to be a significant risk factor. Until recently, true fallopian tube cancers were very rare. The historic requirement for the diagnosis of a fallopian tube cancer included the following: (1) the main tumor is grossly in the fallopian tube; (2) microscopically, the mucosa is chiefly involved and has a papillary pattern; and (3) if the tubal wall is involved to a great extent, the transition between benign and malignant tubal epithelium should be demonstrated [2]. Truthfully, many serous "ovarian cancers" probably do begin elsewhere and metastasize to the ovary since ovarian stromal involvement is the principle requirement to categorize a malignancy as primary ovarian cancer. Since serous peritoneal, fallopian tube, and ovarian cancers are histologically and morphologically similar regardless of where they begin, and are treated alike, they have been collectively categorized as ovarian cancer. Today, our approach to treatment is based on this premise, specifically that all these cancers are lumped together as one. National collaborative group trials for ovarian cancer have typically studied all three malignancies together rather than individually, even non-serous cell types. And this was very sensible, since we thought of ovarian cancer in terms of its anatomic origin and combining made practical sense for clinical trial accrual. This dilemma is apropos given the current belief that the fallopian tube (serous tubal intraepithelial carcinoma, STIC) may be the primary culprit in the etiology of many serous cancers of the ovary [3]. It is very helpful to know what the target is, not just for purposes of tidiness and taxonomy, but also for understanding how to envision the next generation of diagnostic tests.

Kurman and coauthors recently described the need for a paradigm shift in our understanding of ovarian cancer [4]. Endometrial precursors are likely responsible for many of the Type I ovarian cancers as endometrioid and clear cell types originate ostensibly from endometriotic implants. These are typically indolent, low-grade malignancies, and endometrioid, transitional and clear cell cancers with distinct molecular markers: KRAS, BRAF, ERB-2, PTEN and others, but not TP-53. And most gastrointestinal-type tumors involving the ovary are also secondary malignancies, with primary mucinous ovarian cancers comprising only 3% of all epithelial ovarian cancers. Fallopian tube precursors are likely the cause of the more common Type II, high-grade serous ovarian cancers which are characterized by TP-53 mutations. In the end, stromal and germ cell tumors may be the only true anatomic ovarian malignancies. The challenge of course, is that all gynecologic cancers are not organ-specific, so our diagnostic and treatment strategies need to evolve.

1. Past

The biomarker past was an era of single-marker diagnostics. CEA was first described in 1965 as a serum biomarker for mucinous colon cancer, and in 1976 as a blood test for women with ovarian cancer [1,5]. At the time, this was a tremendous advance in science. Not long after, cancer antigen 125 (CA125) was announced as a serum biomarker specific for ovarian cancer [6] (Table 1). To move from an age of very limited imaging and diagnostics to an ovarian cancer blood test was transformational. In retrospect, it can be argued that CA125 has done little to improve ovarian cancer care. The Food and Drug Administration (FDA) never approved CA125 for preoperative use in the United States, but only for cancer surveillance for women with a known diagnosis of ovarian cancer. Ironically, the majority of CA125 tests ordered today are for the evaluation of an ovarian tumor prior to surgery. The use of serum CA125 has also never been associated with a survival benefit, whether utilized before or after diagnosis. This may be an indictment of the test itself, of the disease, the stage at diagnosis, treatment options, or a combination of these factors.

Table 1. Common serum biomarkers for ovarian cancer, year of publication or Food and Drug Administration (FDA) clearance. CEA, carcinoembyonic antigen; CA125, cancer antigen 125; ROMA, Risk of Ovarian Malignancy Algorithm; HE4, human epididymis protein 4; Ova1 and Overa are proprietary multivariate index assays, Vermillion, Inc.

Biomarker	Year
CEA	1965
CA125	1981
HE4	2008
Ova1	2009
ROMA	2010
Overa	2016

Although CA125 is the best-known serum ovarian cancer biomarker, it is not the only one: CEA (mucinous), LDH (dysgerminoma, mixed germ cell tumors), β-hCG (choriocarcinoma, mixed germ cell tumors), inhibin B (granulosa cell tumors), α-fetoprotein (yolk sac tumors, embryonal cell tumors), and HE4 are also available. In 2008, HE4 was cleared by the FDA for use in monitoring patients with a known diagnosis of ovarian cancer, able to detect recurrence of epithelial cancers 2 to 3 months in advance of CA125. Like CA125, it does not have a preoperative diagnostic indication from the FDA. CA125 is the most studied biomarker for serous epithelial cancer arising from the ovary, fallopian tube, or peritoneal cavity, but it is neither a sensitive nor particularly specific cancer marker. This may partly explain why its use has not translated into an improvement in patient survival. For 35 years, we have been trying to overcome this biomarker's inadequacy by combining it with other markers, combining it with imaging, or monitoring its behavior over time: all ultimately without epic success. Success, our patients have discovered, is identifying ovarian cancer in the earliest of stages where treatment can have a lasting impact on survival. Our understanding of protein biomarkers has improved recently as a result of advances in proteomic diagnostic technologies.

2. Present

In 2009, the FDA cleared the first preoperative serum biomarker test for ovarian cancer. After five years of diagnostic discovery and systematic clinical testing, a 5-protein biomarker panel named Ova1® became the first multivariate index assay (MIA) to gain clearance in the United States [7,8]. Ova1 combines the second generation CA125-II with other inflammatory and transport proteins (transferrin, β-2 microglobulin, apolipoprotein A-1, and transthyretin) into a test result of low or high risk for ovarian cancer. The following year, a two-protein test was FDA-cleared that combined CA125 and HE4 (Risk of Ovarian Malignancy Algorithm, ROMA®) for identical indications [9]. These MIA tests were a significant improvement for preoperative testing compared to single biomarker tests because of increased sensitivity (Table 2) [10]. Importantly, these tests are not true diagnostic tests, but rather triage or referral tests. When a woman is known to have an ovarian tumor that requires surgery, these tests are used to determine the likelihood of malignancy. A primary care provider can utilize the test to determine whether referral to a gynecologic oncologist is indicated. These tests have two critical requirements: (1) a mass has been confirmed on imaging, and (2) the ovarian tumor has already been determined to require surgery. Since the test itself is not used to determine whether or not surgery is necessary, it should result in minimal tangible harm. Nationwide, the majority of ovarian cancer surgeries are not initially performed by a gynecologic oncologist, so the hope is that the quality of patient care and cancer survival will improve over time as appropriate referrals are made. Provided that the two critical requirements are observed, this carefully considered strategy should prevent unnecessary surgery from a falsely positive biomarker test, an important consideration for the women, their doctors, and the FDA.

Table 2. Test performance for detecting ovarian cancer of all histologic types.

Biomarker	Sensitivity	Specificity
CA125 *,+,#	76%	94%
Oval *	94%	54%
ROMA ^	89%	83%
Overa *	91%	69%

* Studied in same patient population; + CA125-II assay (second generation); # CA125 not FDA-approved for preoperative use; ^ Meta-analysis [11]

Multivariate index assays have continued to evolve. In 2016, the FDA cleared a new generation Oval test (Overa®) that essentially combines two MIA tests and maintains a high diagnostic sensitivity with improved specificity [12], Table 2. The individual markers are CA125-II, HE4, apolipoprotein A-1, follicle stimulating hormone, and transferrin. The preoperative indications are the same. Other panels will soon follow [13]. Naturally, there are always temptations to move a diagnostic test into a screening role, but without proper study, this is a premature and potentially harmful notion. Cancer screening and cancer diagnostics are vastly different challenges with regard to disease prevalence and endpoint objectives.

Ovarian biomarkers are not restricted to the blood. Ultrasound, like all imaging, is a biomarker of disease. Ultrasound has been widely studied in the United States and Europe as a screening tool and as a diagnostic adjunct. We are beginning to discover that ovarian ultrasound screening alone, or in combination with CA125, may have the potential to save lives [14,15]. Findings from the United Kingdom Collaborative Trial of Ovarian Cancer Screening (UKCTOCS) recently reported preliminary results of a shift to early stage disease and a reduction in cancer deaths on follow up to 14 years with multimodal ovarian cancer screening with serum CA125 interpreted using the Risk of Ovarian Cancer Algorithm (ROCA), transvaginal ultrasound, and clinical assessment. ROCA is an algorithm used to interpret longitudinal CA125 values for ovarian cancer screening. This story is far from over, but it is definitely premature to begin screening the general population off protocol. In fact, shortly following the UKCTOCS publication, the FDA, the American College of Obstetrics and Gynecology, and the Society of Gynecologic Oncology all made prompt safety statements announcing that ROCA is not an approved screening strategy and may trigger unnecessary surgical procedures.

How we combine biomarkers has a significant impact on their overall test performance. Tests can be combined in series or parallel. When combined in series (A, B and C, etc.), the statistical consequence is improved specificity at the expense of sensitivity. Conversely, tests combined in parallel (A or B or C, etc.) will result in improved sensitivity with a compromise in specificity. At the risk of oversimplification, the MIA tests are essentially combining individual biomarker tests in a parallel manner. Ova1 is a good example. Five biomarkers are applied in parallel in the same serum specimen with resultant high sensitivity (and high negative predictive value), making it an excellent triage test. If the test is low-risk, it is very unlikely to be malignant and the patient can have surgery without consulting a specialist. But the apparent drawback of this MIA strategy can be a modest specificity and ovarian tumors may have a high-risk test result even though cancer is not present. By requiring that a mass be confirmed on imaging prior to ordering Ova1, there is a mandate of sorts to combine an additional test (imaging) that localizes the problem to the ovary, improving both the sensitivity of finding an abnormality and the specificity that the problem arises from the ovary (though not that it is necessarily malignant).

Today, serum biomarkers alone are not enough. In developed countries, there is no practical way to divorce serum biomarkers from ovarian imaging since ultrasound and CT scan are ubiquitous tests available to nearly every woman. Ultrasound is far less expensive than a CT scan or MRI, but ultrasound findings are limited mainly to the pelvis. An ultrasound-based morphology scoring system is an effective and objective way to identify ovarian tumors at high-risk for malignancy. The International Ovarian Tumor Analysis group (IOTA) has a multifaceted algorithm that has been systematically evaluated in Europe to high acclaim [16]. There have also been attempts to simplify the IOTA algorithm [17,18], and IOTA has yet to be evaluated in the United States. Other morphology-based indices have been proposed and validated in the U.S. and abroad [19–21]. Moreover, much like longitudinal CA125 (ROCA), serial ultrasound offers improved diagnostic results over a single evaluation (Figure 1) [22,23]. Serial ultrasonography is a sensible approach because each tumor is evaluated both on its changing complexity and its physiologic evolution. There can be clinical reasons not to perform serial evaluations on women with ovarian tumors. First, the presentation may be so concerning for malignancy that prompt surgery is best. Second, the woman may be symptomatic from the tumor so delayed intervention is problematic. Third, the patient may be traveling a great distance or have other personal reasons why a delay in treatment is not feasible. In the absence of these issues, a thoughtful re-evaluation is a valuable diagnostic option, and the data support this concept for serum CA125 in ovarian cancer screening (ROCA) and serial ultrasound with a quantifiable morphology index score in ovarian diagnostics (and maybe screening). The coup de gras, given our present diagnostic capability, would be a combination of serial MIA biomarkers with serial ultrasound. This data has yet to be published.

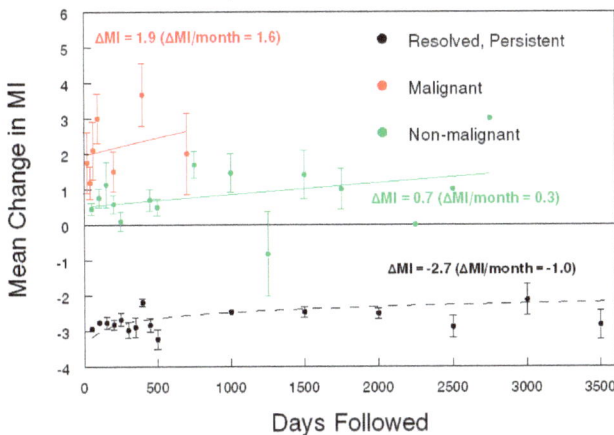

Figure 1. Results of serial ultrasound evaluation of ovarian tumors. MI, Morphology Index score, University of Kentucky (Lexington, KY, USA).

3. Yet-To-Come

Dickens was artful in his portrayal of Ebenezer Scrooge, allowing him to see his unflattering future through Marley's ghost of Christmas yet-to-come. Of course, after his apparitional vision on Christmas Eve, Scrooge awoke transformed. And transformation is what we need for ovarian cancer diagnostics. It is certainly possible that new innovations will give rise to novel diagnostic insights, just as cancer therapy is trending toward targeted, molecular-based treatment. Although personalized cancer treatment is still far from the standard of care, it does raise the question, "Can we pursue a similar evolution in ovarian cancer diagnostics?" After 50 years, it is regrettable that we are still searching for effective approaches to early cancer diagnosis, but we are. As we transition our thinking and our oncology research to a molecular genetic model, we will recognize that this will unite malignancies in a different way, based on common molecular footprints rather than on an anatomic location or a given oncology specialty.

In the near term, we will see new types of serum cancer biomarkers that outperform our current protein-based markers in both selectivity and accuracy. Nucleic acids are showing promise as a new group of serum markers, including free DNA, mRNA, microRNAs, and circulating tumor DNA (ctDNA) [24,25]. A thoughtful combination of protein and nucleic acid markers may permit a comprehensive screening and diagnostic panel that captures all gynecologic malignancies in one blood test. In the future, an annual pelvic ultrasound and a comprehensive serum biomarker screening/diagnostic panel may replace the much maligned bimanual examination as part of the annual gynecologic examination. If abnormal, repeat testing will provide a personalized, serial database that will recalculate the likelihood of malignancy based on the objective change over time in tumor morphology and physiology. As the diagnosis and treatment of cancer changes, so too must clinical trial design to accommodate the new era of multiple biomarkers and targeted, personalized therapies [26].

Beyond the near future, germ-line cancer testing will be initiated at birth as part of newborn screening. Today, we often recommend genetic cancer testing following a malignant diagnosis, which is helpful for their future screening and for their relatives, but it is obviously a little late to prevent their own cancer. The power of knowing individual genetic risk at birth is that it may potentially modify behavior in those found to have a germ-line mutation, which comprise 5%–10% of cancers, and permit selective screening algorithms that are customized to personal cancer risk. And periodic genomic screening throughout one's lifetime may help identify acquired mutations that predispose to specific cancers, heighten awareness, alter personal behavior, and dictate medical surveillance. The technology to sort, store and personalize this colossal amount of data is available today, a consequence of Moore's law whereby computer processing speeds and power have roughly doubled every two years beginning in the 1960s. Cancer testing will quickly move beyond organ and specialty-specific screening. Whole body scans and universal cancer panels will screen and monitor all cancers, solid and hematogenous. An asymptomatic patient may not even need to see a physician if the annual evaluation is normal. A new medical field for screening and early diagnostics will emerge for physicians and epidemiologists, a field of study that is independent of patient gender, organ, or the subspecialties of today.

To get there, we must agree to work with industry innovators in medicine, technology and finance to develop and fund novel strategies for diagnosis and screening. We must encourage the national collaborative groups and the National Cancer Institute's Clinical Trials Reporting Program to promote screening and diagnostic trials with as much vigor as the interventional treatment trials. Since the early detection of any cancer has the promise of shifting diagnosis to an earlier stage, cancer survival will improve. This approach could ultimately revolutionize how we provide care for our patients, and perhaps spare us yet another salvage chemotherapy trial for relapsed ovarian cancer.

So let us awake on a future Christmas morning with newfound clarity. Let us transform how we categorize ovarian cancer, how we identify ovarian cancer, how we treat ovarian cancer, and possibly how we screen for cancer in general. It did not take long for the Nuclear Age to change our worldview or for the Information Age to profoundly alter our daily lives; with any luck, it will not take long to revisit our approach to early diagnostics for ovarian cancer. If Ebenezer Scrooge can change his ways …

Conflicts of Interest: The author declare no conflict of interest.

References

1. Gold, P.; Freedman, S. Demonstration of tumor-specific antigens in human colonic carcinomata by immunological tolerance and absorption techniques. *J. Exp. Med.* **1965**, *121*, 439–462. [CrossRef] [PubMed]
2. Hu, C.; Taymor, M.; Hertig, A. Primary carcinoma of the fallopian tube. *Am. J. Obstet. Gynecol.* **1950**, *59*, 58–67. [CrossRef]
3. Kindelberger, D.; Miron, L.; Hirsch, M.; Feltmate, C.; Medeiros, F.; Callahan, M.; Garner, E.; Gordon, R.; Birch, C.; Berkowitz, R.; et al. Intraepithelial carcinoma of the fimbria and pelvic serous carcinoma: Evidence for a causal relationship. *Am. J. Surg. Pathol.* **2007**, *2*, 161–169. [CrossRef] [PubMed]
4. Kurman, R.; Shih, I. Molecular pathogenesis and extraovarian origin of epithelial ovarian cancer—Shifting the paradigm. *Hum. Pathol.* **2011**, *7*, 918–931. [CrossRef] [PubMed]
5. Khoo, S.; MacKay, E. Carcinoembryonic antigen (CEA) in ovarian cancer: Factors influencing its incidence and changes which occur in response to cytotoxic drugs. *Br. J. Obstet. Gynaecol.* **1976**, *83*, 753–759. [CrossRef] [PubMed]
6. Bast, R.; Feeney, M.; Lazarus, H.; Nadler, L.; Knapp, R. Reactivity of a monoclonal antibody with human ovarian carcinoma. *J. Clin. Investig.* **1981**, *68*, 1331–1337. [CrossRef] [PubMed]
7. Ueland, F.; DeSimone, C.; Seamon, L.; Miller, R.; Goodrich, S.; Podzielinski, I.; Sokoll, L.; Smith, A.; van Nagell, J.R., Jr.; Zhang, Z. Effectiveness of a multivariate index assay in the preoperative assessment of ovarian tumors. *Obstet. Gynecol.* **2011**, *117*, 1289–1297. [CrossRef] [PubMed]
8. Zhang, Z.; Chan, D. The road from discovery to clinical diagnostics: Lessons learned from the first FDA-cleared in vitro diagnostic multivariate index assay of proteomic biomarkers. *Cancer Epidemiol. Biomark. Prev.* **2010**, *19*, 2995–2999. [CrossRef] [PubMed]
9. Moore, R.; Miller, M.; Disilvestro, P.; Landrum, L.; Gajewski, W.; Ball, J.; Skates, S. Evaluation of the diagnostic accuracy of the risk of ovarian malignancy algorithm in women with a pelvic mass. *Obstet. Gynecol.* **2011**, *118*, 280–288. [CrossRef] [PubMed]
10. Bristow, R.; Smith, A.; Zhang, Z.; Chan, D.; Crutcher, G.; Fung, E.; Munroe, D. Ovarian malignancy risk stratification of the adnexal mass using a multivariate index assay. *Gynecol. Oncol.* **2013**, *128*, 252–259. [CrossRef] [PubMed]
11. Li, F.; Tie, R.; Chang, K.; Wang, F.; Deng, S.; Lu, W.; Yu, L.; Chen, M. Does risk for ovarian malignancy algorithm excel human epididymis protein 4 and CA125 in predicting epithelial ovarian cancer: A meta-analysis. *BMC Cancer* **2012**, *12*, 258. [CrossRef] [PubMed]
12. Coleman, R.; Herzog, T.; Chan, D.; Munroe, D.; Pappas, T.; Smith, A.; Zhang, Z.; Wolf, J. Validation of a second-generation multivariate index assay for malignancy risk of adnexal masses. *Am. J. Obstet. Gynecol.* **2016**, *215*, 82.e1–82.e11. [CrossRef] [PubMed]
13. Simmons, A.; Clarke, C.; Badgwell, D.; Lu, Z.; Sokoll, L.; Lu, K.; Zhang, Z.; Bast, R.; Skates, S. Validation of a biomarker panel and longitudinal biomarker performance for early detection of ovarian cancer. *Int. J. Gynecol. Cancer* **2016**, *26*, 1070–1077. [CrossRef] [PubMed]
14. Jacobs, I.; Menon, U.; Ryan, A.; Maharaj, A.; Burnell, M.; Kalsi, J.; Amso, N.; Apostolidou, S.; Benjamin, E.; Cruickshank, D.; et al. Ovarian cancer screening and mortality in the UK Collaborative Trial of Ovarian Cancer Screeening (UKCTOCS): A randomized controlled trial. *Lancet* **2016**, *387*, 945–956. [CrossRef]
15. Ormsby, E.; Pavlik, E.; van Nagell, J. Ultrasound follow up of an adnexal mass has the potential to save lives. *Am. J. Obstet. Gynecol.* **2015**, *213*, 657–661. [CrossRef] [PubMed]
16. Timmerman, D.; van Calster, B.; Testa, A.; Guerriero, S.; Fischerova, D.; Lissoni, A.; van Holsbeke, C.; Fruscio, R.; Czekierdowski, A.; Jurkovic, D.; et al. Ovarian cancer prediction in adnexal masses using ultrasound-based logistic regression models: A temporal and external validation study by the IOTA group. *Ultrasound Obstet. Gynecol.* **2010**, *36*, 226–234. [CrossRef] [PubMed]
17. Timmerman, D.; Testa, A.; Bourne, T.; Ameye, L.; Jurkovic, D.; van Holsbeke, C.; Paladini, D.; van Calster, B.; Vergote, I.; van Huffel, S.; et al. Simple ultrasound-based rules for the diagnosis of ovarian cancer. *Ultrasound Obstet. Gynecol.* **2008**, *31*, 681–690. [CrossRef] [PubMed]

18. Van Caster, B.; van Hoorde, K.; Valentin, L.; Testa, A.; Fischerova, D.; van Holsbeke, C.; Savelli, L.; Franchi, D.; Epstein, E.; Kaijser, J.; et al. Evaluating the risk of ovarian cancer before surgery using the ADNEX model to differentiate between benign, borderline, early and advanced stage invasive, and secondary metastatic tumours: Prospective multicentre diagnostic study. *BMJ* **2014**, *349*, 1–14. [CrossRef] [PubMed]

19. Ueland, F.; DePriest, P.; Pavlik, E.; Kryscio, R.; van Nagell, J., Jr. Preoperative differentiation of malignant from benign ovarian tumors: The efficacy of morphology indexing and Doppler flow sonography. *Gynecol. Oncol.* **2003**, *91*, 46–50. [CrossRef]

20. Barnsfather, K.; Fitzpatrick, C.; Wilson, J.; Linn, C.; Brizendine, E.; Schilder, J. The Morphology Index: Predictive value of malignancy among clinicians at various levels of training. *Gynecol. Oncol.* **2012**, *127*, 94–97. [CrossRef] [PubMed]

21. Jeoung, H.; Choi, H.; Lim, Y.; Lee, M.; Kim, S.; Han, S.; Ahn, T.; Choi, S. The efficacy of sonographic morphology indexing and serum CA-125 for preoperative differentiation of malignant from benign ovarian tumors in patients after operation with ovarian tumors. *J. Gynecol. Oncol.* **2008**, *19*, 229–235. [CrossRef] [PubMed]

22. Elder, J.; Pavlik, E.; Long, A.; Miller, R.; DeSimone, C.; Hoff, J.; Ueland, W.; Kryscio, R.; van Nagell, J.; Ueland, F. Serial ultrasonographic evaluation of ovarian abnormalities with a morphology index. *Gynecol. Oncol.* **2014**, *135*, 8–12. [CrossRef] [PubMed]

23. Pavlik, E.; Ueland, F.; Miller, R.; Ubellacker, J.; DeSimone, C.; Elder, J.; Hoff, J.; Baldwin, L.; Kryscio, R.; van Nagell, J.R., Jr. Frequency and disposition of ovarian abnormalities followed with serial transvaginal sonography. *Obstet. Gynecol.* **2013**, *122*, 210–217. [CrossRef] [PubMed]

24. Schwarzenbach, H.; Hoon, D.; Pantel, K. Cell-free nucleic acids as biomarkers in cancer patients. *Nat. Rev. Cancer* **2011**, *11*, 426–437. [CrossRef] [PubMed]

25. Bettegowda, C.; Sausen, M.; Leary, R.; Kinde, I.; Wang, Y.; Agrawal, N.; Bartlett, B.; Wang, H.; Luber, B.; Alani, R.; et al. Detection of circulating tumor DNA in early- and late-stage human malignancies. *Sci. Transl. Med.* **2014**, *224*, 224ra24. [CrossRef] [PubMed]

26. Venook, A.; Arcila, M.; Benson, A.; Berry, D.; Camidge, D.; Carlson, R.; Choueiri, T.; Guild, V.; Kalemkerian, G.; Kurzrock, R.; et al. NCCN Work Group Report: Designing clinical trials in the era of multiple biomarkers and targeted therapies. *J. Natl. Compr. Cancer Netw.* **2014**, *12*, 1629–1649.

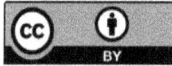

diagnostics

MDPI

Article

Complications from Surgeries Related to Ovarian Cancer Screening

Lauren A. Baldwin, Edward J. Pavlik, Emma Ueland, Hannah E. Brown, Kelsey M. Ladd, Bin Huang, Christopher P. DeSimone, John R. van Nagell, Frederick R. Ueland and Rachel W. Miller *

Division of Gynecologic Oncology, Department of Obstetrics and Gynecology, The University of Kentucky Chandler Medical Center and the Markey Cancer Center, 800 Rose Street, Lexington, KY 40536-0293, USA; labald1@uky.edu (L.A.B.); Epaul1@uky.edu (E.J.P.); emmaueland_2017@depauw.edu (E.U.); hannah.e.brown@duke.edu (H.E.B.); Kelsey.ladd@uky.edu (K.M.L.); bhuang@kcr.uky.edu (B.H.); cpdesi00@uky.edu (C.P.D.); jrvann2@email.uky.edu (J.R.v.N.); fuela0@email.uky.edu (F.R.U.)
* Correspondence: raware00@uky.edu; Tel.: +1-859-323-2169; Fax: +1-859-323-1018

Academic Editor: Andreas Kjaer
Received: 7 December 2016; Accepted: 28 February 2017; Published: 8 March 2017

Abstract: The aim of this study was to evaluate complications of surgical intervention for participants in the Kentucky Ovarian Cancer Screening Program and compare results to those of the Prostate, Lung, Colorectal and Ovarian Cancer Screening trial. A retrospective database review included 657 patients who underwent surgery for a positive screen in the Kentucky Ovarian Cancer Screening Program from 1988–2014. Data were abstracted from operative reports, discharge summaries, and office notes for 406 patients. Another 142 patients with incomplete records were interviewed by phone. Complete information was available for 548 patients. Complications were graded using the Clavien–Dindo (C–D) Classification of Surgical Complications and considered minor if assigned Grade I (any deviation from normal course, minor medications) or Grade II (other pharmacological treatment, blood transfusion). C–D Grade III complications (those requiring surgical, endoscopic, or radiologic intervention) and C–D Grade IV complications (those which are life threatening) were considered "major". Statistical analysis was performed using SAS 9.4 software. Complications were documented in 54/548 (10%) subjects. For women with malignancy, 17/90 (19%) had complications compared to 37/458 (8%) with benign pathology ($p < 0.003$). For non-cancer surgery, obesity was associated with increased complications ($p = 0.0028$). Fifty patients had minor complications classified as C–D Grade II or less. Three of 4 patients with Grade IV complications had malignancy ($p < 0.0004$). In the Prostate, Lung, Colorectal and Ovarian Cancer Screening trial, 212 women had surgery for ovarian malignancy, and 95 had at least one complication (45%). Of the 1080 women with non-cancer surgery, 163 had at least one complication (15%). Compared to the Prostate, Lung, Colorectal and Ovarian Cancer Screening trial, the Kentucky Ovarian Cancer Screening Program had significantly fewer complications from both cancer and non-cancer surgery ($p < 0.0001$ and $p = 0.002$, respectively). Complications resulting from surgery performed as a result of the Kentucky Ovarian Cancer Screening Program were infrequent and significantly fewer than reported in the Prostate, Lung, Colorectal and Ovarian Cancer Screening trial. Complications were mostly minor (93%) and were more common in cancer versus non-cancer surgery.

Keywords: ovarian cancer screening; complications; ovary; cancer; screening

1. Introduction

Ovarian cancer is the most common cause of gynecologic cancer death in the United States with 22,280 new cases and 14,240 deaths from the disease in 2016 [1]. Despite the introduction of targeted therapies, refinements in novel chemotherapy regimens, and advances in surgical techniques, survival outcomes have remained essentially unchanged over time [2]. Most patients with ovarian cancer are diagnosed with advanced stage disease where survival outcomes are poor. Surgical stage at the time of diagnosis remains among the most important prognostic factors for patients with ovarian cancer. Women with Stage I disease, where cancer is confined to one or both ovaries have a 10-year survival rate of 74%, whereas those with Stages II, III, and IV disease have 10-year survival rates of 45%, 21%, and <5%, respectively [3]. Identifying women with early stage disease is difficult since early ovarian cancer does not reliably cause symptoms. A specific symptom profile has been described in patients with ovarian cancer; however, it is most often reported in those with advanced stage disease [4]. Early stage disease rarely demonstrates this symptom profile [5,6].

The key to a successful screening program is the increased detection of early stage disease and subsequent improved survival in the screen-detected cancers. Efforts in ovarian cancer screening have focused on the integration of transvaginal sonography and serum biomarkers, specifically CA 125 [7–10]. Improved survival from ovarian cancer screening has been reported [11–13], especially with regard to screen-detected incident ovarian cancers [9,14]. One large trial (the Prostate, Lung, Colorectal and Ovarian (PLCO) Randomized Controlled Screening Trial: *PLCO trial*) failed to observe improved survival in the intervention (screening) group [15] and reported a surprisingly high false positive rate with 19 women recommended for surgery for every malignancy that was identified [16]. This is in contrast to other screening studies that reported lower false positive rates [9,11,13]. In the PLCO trial, screen positive cases found to be non-malignant at surgery had an unexpectedly high complication rate (15%) [15] and led to announcements that ovarian cancer screening does more harm than good [17]. In comparison, the United Kingdom Controlled Trial on Ovarian Cancer Screening (UKCTOCS trial) reported a surgical complication rate of less than 1% [9].

The present study examines complications in women undergoing surgery as a result of an abnormality detected in the Kentucky Ovarian Cancer Screening Program, an ultrasound-based program that has screened over 40,000 women from 1988 to present. We objectively evaluated the number and type of complications observed in these women using the Clavien–Dindo (C–D) Classification of Surgical Complications [18,19] and compared findings to those reported in the PLCO trial.

2. Methods

The study was approved by the (University of Kentucky Institutional Review Board protocol 88-0021-9F with the most recent renewal on 11 August 2016. Women enrolled in the Kentucky Ovarian Cancer Screening Program from 26 May 1988 to 1 June 2014 were included in the study group (*n* = 41,529). The University of Kentucky Institutional Review Board approved this study. Women were recruited by physician referral, media announcements, and word of mouth. Eligibility criteria included asymptomatic women age 50 years or older without a family history of ovarian cancer, or those 25 years or older with a documented family history of ovarian cancer in at least one first or second-degree relative, and the ability to read and understand the informed consent presented in English. Women under clinical evaluation because of pelvic symptoms, a known ovarian tumor, or a personal history of ovarian cancer were excluded. Women enrolled in the Kentucky Ovarian Cancer Screening Program underwent annual screening with transvaginal sonography. Abnormalities were managed according to the study algorithm (Figure 1), which included increased frequency of screening with transvaginal sonography, assessment of morphology index score, and serum CA 125 (Figure 2). Diagnostic surgical intervention was recommended if results indicated at least moderate risk of malignancy according to the published protocol [20]. Minimally invasive surgical technique was preferred, unless medical issues prohibited this approach. Details of the study algorithm, threshold for intervention, and cancer outcomes have been previously published [12,20].

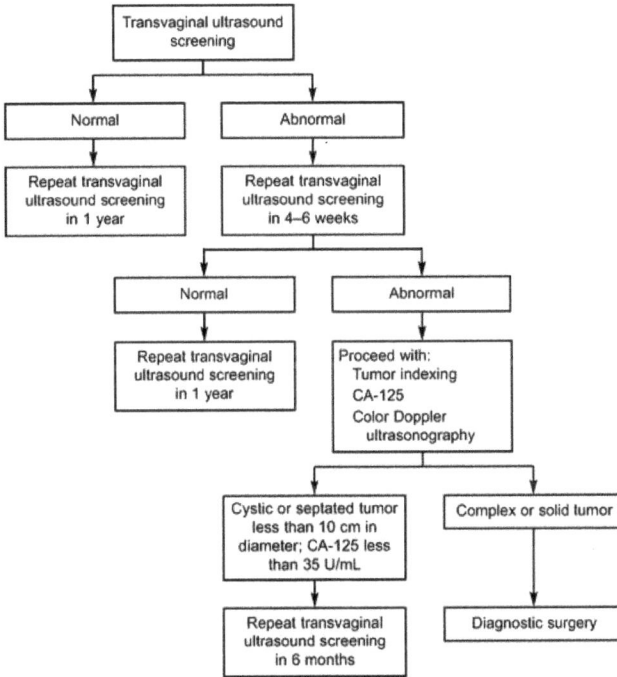

Figure 1. Study algorithm for the Kentucky Ovarian Cancer Screening Program. Reprinted from [12].

Figure 2. Morphology Index (numeric value 0–10). Reprinted from [12].

In the first 26 years of the Kentucky Ovarian Cancer Screening Program, 657 patients underwent surgical intervention for positive screens. Three investigators performed a thorough review of all available medical records including operative reports, discharge summaries, and office notes. Phone interviews were conducted when medical records were incomplete. A complication was defined as any deviation from the normal postoperative course within 60 days of surgery. Complete information was obtained for 548 patients. Physician investigators graded all surgical complications that were identified in these 548 patients according to the C–D Classification of Surgical Complications (Table 1) [18,19]. Complications were considered "minor" if they were C–D Grades I or II. Grade I complications included any minor deviations from a normal postoperative course without the need for pharmacologic intervention. Grade II complications consisted of complications treated pharmacologically. C–D Grade III complications (those requiring surgical, endoscopic, or radiologic intervention) and C–D Grade IV complications (those which are life threatening) were considered "major."

Table 1. Classification of Surgical Complications. Modified from [19].

C–D Grades	Definition
Grade I	Any deviation from normal postoperative course without the need for pharmacological treatment or surgical, endoscopic and radiological interventions. Acceptable therapeutic regimens are: drugs as antiemetics, antipyretics, analgetics, diuretics, and electrolytes and physiotherapy.
Grade II	Requiring pharmacological treatment with drugs other thanthan such allowed for Grade I complications.
Grade III	Requiring surgical, endoscopic or radiologic intervention.
Grade III-a	Intervention not under general anesthesia.
Grade III-b	Intervention under general anesthesia.
Grade IV	Life threatening complications (including CNS complications) ‡ requiring IC/ICU management.
Grade IV-a	Single organ dysfunction (including dialysis).
Grade IV-b	Multi organ dysfunction.
Grade V	Death of patient.
Suffix "d"	If the patient suffers from a complication at the time of discharge (see examples in Appendix B, http://Links.Lww.com/SLA/A3), the suffix "d" (for "disability") is added to the respective grade of complication. This label indicates the need for a follow-up to fully evaluate the complication.

‡ Brain hemorrhage, ischemic stroke, subarachnoid bleeding, but excluding transient ischemic attacks (TIA); IC: intermediate care; ICU: intensive care unit (www.surgicalcomplications.info).

Descriptive analysis for demographics and clinical factors was performed. We used χ^2 tests to examine associations between complication status (yes and no) and other factors such as age, race, body mass index (BMI), type of surgery, cancer status, and type of hospital where surgery was performed. Multivariate logistic regressions were fitted to evaluate the association between complication status and other factors. The final model included only covariates with a significance level of 0.05 or less. Model goodness of fit, multicollinearity, and interactions were also examined. All analyses were performed using SAS Statistical software version 9.4. All statistical tests were two-sided with a p-value ≤ 0.05 used to identify statistical significance.

3. Results

Complete clinical information was available on 548 of the 657 patients who underwent surgery for positive screens in the Kentucky Ovarian Cancer Screening Program between the years of 1988–2014. A summary of demographic information is presented in Table 2 and shows that women with and without complications were similar. Complications were documented in 54 of 548 (10%) subjects. Fifty patients (93%) had minor complications classified as C–D Grade II or less, while four had complications categorized as C–D Grade IV. Complication profiles for individuals are shown relative to age and BMI in Figure 3.

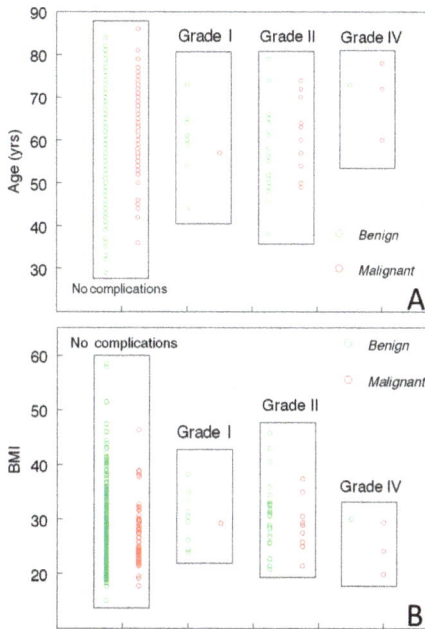

Figure 3. Clavien–Dindo classification of complication relative to age (**A**) and BMI (**B**) in women with benign (**green** circles) and malignant results (**red** circles) at surgery.

Table 2. Demographics of the group studied.

Variable	No Complications	Complications	Excluded
	$N = 494$	$N = 54$	$N = 109$
Age	59.7, 59 (29–86)	59.6, 59 (38–79)	59.6, 60 (36–84)
Weight	163.6, 158.5 (80–368)	173.7, 170 (121–274)	159.2, 150 (101–250)
Height	64.6, 64.5 (55–71)	64.4, 65 (60–70)	64.5, 64 (57–72)
BMI	27.6, 26.6 (15.1–58.4)	29.4, 29.2 (19.9–45.7)	26.9, 25.8 (18–43.9)
Family history of:			
Ovarian cancer	132 (26.7%)	15 (27.8%)	36 (33%)
Breast cancer	27 (50%)	217 (43.9%)	46 (42.2%)
Breast cancer personal history	8 (14.8%)	39 (7.9%)	8 (7.3%)
Colon cancer	128 (25.9%)	11 (20.3%)	46 (24.7%)
Colon cancer personal history	3 (0.6%)	0 (0%)	1 (0.9%)
No history of hormone replacement therapy	372 (75.3%)	43 (79.6%)	65 (59.6%)
History of hormone replacement therapy	122 (24.7%)	11 (20.4%)	38 (34.9%)
Menopausal Status			
Premenopausal	73 (14.8%)	6 (11.1%)	18 (16.5%)
Perimenopausal	18 (3.6%)	0	7 (6.4%)
Postmenopausal	403 (81.6%)	48 (88.9%)	84 (77.1%)
Any symptoms	254 (51%)	30 (55.5%)	51 (46.8%)
Ovarian cancer symptoms *	27 (14.8%)	4 (7.4%)	5 (4.6%)
Other symptoms **	248 (50.2%)	30 (55.6%	48 (44%)

Mean, median (range) * Women reporting pelvic or abdominal pain, being unable to eat normally, feeling full quickly, feeling abdominal bloating or increased abdominal size presenting for >12 days per month with an onset in less than the last 12 months. ** Women reporting back pain, indigestion, nausea, vomiting, weight loss, urinary urgency, frequent urination, constipation, menstrual irregularities, bleeding after menopause, pain during intercourse, fatigue, leg swelling, difficulty breathing. Any symptoms: any symptom included under ovarian cancer symptoms or other symptoms without regard to frequency of duration.

Complication rates were compared for surgeries that resulted in the diagnosis of malignancy versus surgery for false positive screens with benign pathology. For women with malignancy, 17 of 90 (19%) had complications compared to 37 of 458 (8%) with benign pathology ($p < 0.003$), Figure 4. Thus, a diagnosis of cancer increased the likelihood of complications with an odds ratio of 2.65. Three of four patients with C–D Grade IV complications had malignancy, while one Grade IV complications occurred in the benign conditions group ($p < 0.0004$). In the PLCO trial, 212 women in the intervention group had surgery for ovarian malignancy, and 95 had at least one complication (45%). Of the 1080 women with surgery with a benign outcome, 163 had at least one complication (15%), yielding an odds ratio of 3 for complications in surgical cancer cases over benign surgical cases. Complication rates from the Kentucky Ovarian Cancer Screening Program were compared with the PLCO trial results. Compared to the PLCO trial, the Kentucky Ovarian Cancer Screening Program had significantly fewer complications from both cancer ($p < 0.001$) and non-cancer surgery ($p = 0.002$) based on chi-square analysis (Figure 4).

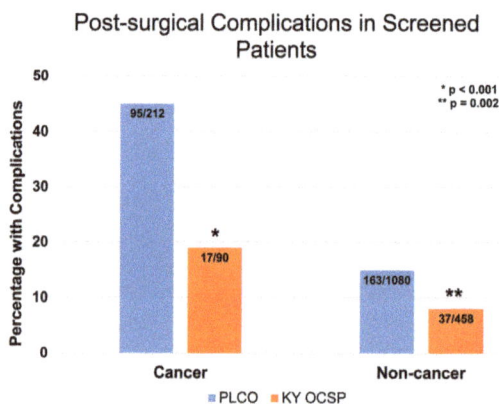

Figure 4. Complications associated with surgery.

Bivariate analysis of complication status versus other clinical variables was performed and obesity was associated with increased incidence of complication, $p = 0.049$ (Table 3). Evaluating clinical variables by cancer status, obesity was not associated with increased complications in surgeries performed for non-cancer pathology, $p = 0.458$ (Table 4). While patients with a cancer diagnosis were significantly older than those with a benign diagnosis, $p = 0.002$ (Table 4), age was not different for those who had complications when compared to those that did not, $p = 0.463$ (Table 3). Other factors evaluated in bivariate analysis did not show significant differences based on complication status.

Table 3. Associations between complications and other factors.

Variables	Complications		No Complications		*p*-Value
	N	%	N	%	
Age					0.463
<50	7	13.0	75	15.2	
50–64	32	59.3	257	52.0	
65–74	10	18.5	121	24.5	
75+	3	5.6	35	7.1	
Unknown	2	3.7	6	1.2	
Weight					0.049
Under-weight	0	0.0	5	1.0	
Normal	11	20.4	185	37.4	
Over-weight	20	37.0	175	35.4	
Obese	20	37.0	108	21.9	
Extreme obesity	3	5.6	21	4.3	

Table 4. Patient characteristics by cancer status.

Variables	Cancer		Non-Cancer		*p*-Value
	N	%	N	%	
Age					0.002
<50	6	6.7	76	16.6	
50–64	38	42.2	251	54.8	
65–74	33	36.7	98	21.4	
75+	11	12.2	27	5.9	
Unknown	2	2.2	6	1.3	
C–D Grade	N	%	N	%	<0.001
None	73	81.1	421	92.0	
Minor	14	15.6	36	7.9	
Severe	3	3.3	1	0.2	
Weight					0.458
Under-weight	1	1.1	4	0.9	
Normal	37	41.1	159	34.7	
Over-weight	31	34.4	164	35.8	
Obese	20	22.2	108	23.6	
Extreme obesity	1	1.1	23	5.0	

In multivariate analysis, obesity was determined to be associated with increased risk of complication versus normal weight (OR 3.17, 1.46–6.90). The location where the procedures were performed was also significantly associated with complication risk (OR 1.97, 1.07–3.65) (Table 5).

Table 5. Odds ratio estimates.

Effect	Odds Ratio	95% Confidence Limits
Age		
Unknown vs. 50–64	4.75	(0.86–26.19)
<50 vs. 50–64	0.76	(0.32–1.81)
75+ vs. 50–64	0.77	(0.22–2.71)
65–74 vs. 50–64	0.69	(0.33–1.48)
Weight		
Overweight vs. Underweight/Normal	2.06	(0.95–4.49)
Obese vs. Underweight/Normal	3.17	(1.46–6.90)
Location		
UK vs. Non-UK	1.97	(1.07–3.65)

4. Discussion

Ovarian cancer is the second most common gynecologic cancer, but the most common cause of gynecologic cancer death. Most women have advanced disease at the time of their diagnosis, with cancer spread throughout the peritoneal cavity and occasionally into the pleural cavity. Despite aggressive surgery and chemotherapy [21], the five-year overall survival for patients with advanced ovarian cancer is less than 30%. Unfortunately, only about 25% of women present with early stage ovarian cancer, where the five-year overall survival may exceed 80%–90% with appropriate surgical staging and adjuvant therapy.

Ovarian cancer screening with transvaginal sonography and serum biomarkers has been explored as a means for increasing the number of women diagnosed with early stage disease [7–13,20]. This shift in stage at diagnosis should result in an improved overall survival as a result of screening. There is a need for ovarian cancer screening because early stage disease rarely produces reliable symptoms. Goff and colleagues reported a symptom profile associated with ovarian cancer [4,22], which included abdominal pain or bloating, pelvic pain, and urinary symptoms present for more than two weeks out of the month and persisting for fewer than 12 months. The effectiveness of a symptom profile is limited as a screening tool because the profile is most useful for identifying advanced stage disease.

Ovarian cancer screening presents unique challenges that are inherent to the disease itself. First, ovarian cancer has a low incidence with only 22,280 new cases expected in 2016, compared to breast or colorectal cancer in women with 246,660 and 68,830 new cases, respectively [1]. The annual balance of deaths from disease to incident cases for ovarian cancer (0.639) is 3.9 times higher than for breast (0.164) and 1.8 times higher than for colorectal cancer (0.346), indicating that ovarian cancer is a much deadlier disease. This is reflected in the low prevalence of ovarian cancer with an estimated 195,767 women living with the disease in the United States in 2013, relative to colorectal (1,177,556) and breast cancers (3,053,450) [23].

A second challenge in ovarian cancer screening is the lack of a thorough understanding of the etiology and natural history of ovarian, primary peritoneal, and fallopian tube cancer. Historically, ovarian cancer was thought to arise from the surface epithelium of the ovary. However, this did not explain normal size ovaries as seen in primary peritoneal cancers. The similarities between serous ovarian and primary peritoneal cancers from the standpoint of genetic mutations, histology, behavior, and response to treatment suggest similar etiologic factors. More recently, investigators have hypothesized that ovarian, primary peritoneal, and fallopian tube cancers originate from serous intraepithelial carcinomas in the fallopian tube [24–33]. If this is the case, then screening for abnormalities of the ovary with transvaginal sonography will prove futile because the early abnormalities exist in the fallopian tube. This model is founded on the presence of microscopic disease that is below the resolution of biomarkers and ultrasonography, and consequently implies that these screening tools cannot be effective. However, the discovery of Stage I cancers in several screening studies indicates that biomarker and ultrasonography screening modalities are sufficiently effective in detecting ovarian cancer early enough to decrease mortality and increase survival [9–12]. Thus, cases that have progressed beyond microscopic disease in the distal fallopian tube can be detected by biomarker and ultrasonography screening often enough to achieve a favorable prognosis for extending survival.

In the present report, we evaluate the complications related to surgery for a positive ovarian cancer screen. In other cancers, such as breast, colon, and cervical, a diagnostic biopsy is performed to determine the presence or absence of malignancy. Percutaneous or transvaginal biopsy of ovarian abnormalities is not recommended because of concern for "seeding" the needle track in the case of malignancy, or for rupturing a malignant tumor, resulting in potentially worse outcomes. Given the aggressive nature of ovarian cancer, these two possibilities could impact the need for adjuvant treatment, or increase the risk of recurrence in early stage disease. As a result, patients with a positive screen indicating a moderate to high risk of malignancy are offered definitive surgery for diagnosis. In most cases, removal of an ovary or ovaries because of an abnormality detected on ovarian cancer screening can be accomplished using a minimally invasive technique, but there are situations when this is not medically recommended. Surgical exploration for a positive screen introduces the possibility of intervention for benign or false positive ovarian abnormalities. The combination of a high percentage of surgeries for women without a malignancy in the PLCO trial (1 malignancy for every 19 surgeries) coupled with a high complication rate [15] led to published statements that screening is harmful [17].

In conclusion, little has been published regarding the nature of the complications reported from surgeries resulting from ovarian cancer screening. In this investigation, we report a low complication rate, with 93% classified as minor. Similarly, the UKCTOCS trial reported a very low complication rate of less than one percent in both screening groups [9]. The procedures of the PLCO trial were to notify the referring physician that a screen was abnormal, but not to make recommendations on whether surgery should be performed or by whom. It is possible that the high complication rates reported in the PLCO trial [15] are related to the recent recognition that better outcomes are achieved when ovarian cancer is treated by specialists at high volume hospitals [34–39], and this benefit may particularly apply to early stage ovarian cancers [40]. Ultimately, the methods used to decide who went to surgery and who would perform the operation may best explain the high false positive rates and high complication rates observed in the PLCO trial.

Acknowledgments: This work was supported by grants from the Telford Foundation, and the Department of Health and Human Services, Commonwealth of Kentucky. Bin Huang received support from the NCI Cancer Center Support Grant (P30 CA177558). No support was received to publish in open access.

Author Contributions: Lauren A. Baldwin contributed to data collection, review and grading of complications, abstract composition and original manuscript composition; Edward J. Pavlik contributed to data collection and manuscript composition; Emma Ueland, Hannah E. Brown, Kelsey M. Ladd contributed to data collection; Bin Huang performed statistical analysis and contributed to manuscript preparation; Christopher P. DeSimone, John R. van Nagell, Frederick R. Ueland contributed to manuscript preparation; and Rachel W. Miller developed the project concept and contributed to data collection, review and grading of complications, and manuscript composition.

Conflicts of Interest: The authors declare no conflicts of interest.

References

1. Siegel, R.L.; Miller, K.D.; Jemal, A. Cancer Statistics. *CA Cancer J. Clin.* **2016**, *66*, 7–30. [CrossRef] [PubMed]
2. Bookman, M.A. Optimal primary therapy of ovarian cancer. *Ann. Oncol.* **2016**, *27*, i58–i62. [CrossRef] [PubMed]
3. Jelovac, D.; Armstrong, D.K. Recent progress in the diagnosis and treatment of ovarian Cancer. *CA Cancer J. Clin.* **2011**, *61*, 183–203. [CrossRef] [PubMed]
4. Goff, B.A.; Mandel, L.S.; Drescher, C.W.; Urban, N.; Gough, S.; Schurman, K.M.; Patras, J.; Mahony, B.S.; Andersen, M.R. Development of an ovarian cancer symptom index. *Cancer* **2007**, *109*, 221–227. [CrossRef] [PubMed]
5. Pavlik, E.J.; Saunders, B.A.; Doran, S.; McHugh, K.W.; Ueland, F.R.; DeSimone, C.P.; DePriest, P.D.; Ware, R.A.; Kryscio, R.J.; van Nagell, J.R. The search for meaning-symptoms and transvaginal sonography screening for ovarian cancer: Predicting malignancy. *Cancer* **2009**, *115*, 3689–3698. [CrossRef] [PubMed]
6. Rossing, M.A.; Wicklund, K.G.; Cushing-Haugen, K.L.; Weiss, N.S. Predictive value of symptoms for early detection of ovarian cancer. *J. Natl. Cancer Inst.* **2010**, *102*, 222–229. [CrossRef] [PubMed]
7. Van Nagell, J.R., Jr.; Pavlik, E.J. Ovarian cancer screening. *Clin. Obstet. Gynecol.* **2012**, *55*, 43–51. [CrossRef] [PubMed]
8. Pavlik, E.J.; Nagell, J.R., Jr. Early detection of ovarian tumors using ultrasound. *Women's Health* **2013**, *9*, 39–55. [CrossRef] [PubMed]
9. Jacobs, I.J.; Menon, U.; Ryan, A.; Gentry-Maharaj, A.; Burnell, M.; Kalsi, J.K.; Amso, N.N.; Apostolidou, S.; Benjamin, E.; Cruickshank, D.; et al. Ovarian cancer screening and mortality in the UK collaborative trial of ovarian cancer screening (UKCTOCS): A randomized controlled trial. *Lancet* **2016**, *387*, 945–956. [CrossRef]
10. Pavlik, E. Ovarian cancer screening effectiveness: A realization from the UKCTOCS. *Women's Health* **2016**, *12*, 475–479. [PubMed]
11. Kobayashi, H.; Yamada, Y.; Sado, T.; Sakata, M.; Yoshida, S.; Kawaguchi, R.; Kanayama, S.; Shigetomi, H.; Haruta, S.; Tsuji, Y.; et al. A randomized study of screening for ovarian cancer: A multicenter study in Japan. *Int. J. Gynecol. Cancer* **2008**, *18*, 414–420. [CrossRef] [PubMed]
12. Van Nagell, J.R., Jr.; Miller, R.W.; DeSimone, C.P.; Ueland, F.R.; Podzielinski, I.; Goodrich, S.T.; Elder, J.W.; Huang, B.; Kryscio, R.J.; Pavlik, E.J. Long-term survival of women with epithelial ovarian cancer detected by ultrasonographic screening. *Obstet. Gynecol.* **2011**, *118*, 1212–1221. [CrossRef] [PubMed]
13. Pavlik, E.J.; Ueland, F.R.; Miller, R.W.; Ubellacker, J.M.; Desimone, C.P.; Elder, J.; Hoff, J.; Baldwin, L.; Kryscio, R.J.; Nagell, J.R., Jr. Frequency and disposition of ovarian abnormalities followed with serial transvaginal ultrasonography. *Obstet. Gynecol.* **2013**, *122*, 210–217. [CrossRef] [PubMed]
14. Jacobs, I.J.; Parmar, M.; Skates, S.J.; Menon, U. Ovarian cancer screening: UKCTOCS trial—Authors' reply. *Lancet* **2016**, *387*, 2603–2604. [CrossRef]
15. Buys, S.S.; Partridge, E.; Black, A.; Johnson, C.C.; Lamerato, L.; Isaacs, C.; Reding, D.J.; Greenlee, R.T.; Yokochi, L.A.; Kessel, B.; et al. Effect of screening on ovarian cancer mortality—The Prostate, Lung, Colorectal and Ovarian (PLCO) Cancer Screening Randomized Controlled Trial. *JAMA* **2011**, *305*, 2295–2303. [CrossRef] [PubMed]
16. Partridge, E.; Greenlee, R.T.; Xu, J.L.; Kreimer, A.R.; Williams, C.; Riley, T.; Reding, D.J.; Church, T.R.; Kessel, B.; Johnson, C.C.; et al. Results from four rounds of ovarian cancer screening in a randomized trial. *Obstet. Gynecol.* **2009**, *113*, 775–782. [CrossRef] [PubMed]

17. Slomski, A. Screening women for ovarian cancer still does more harm than good. *JAMA* **2012**, *307*, 2474–2475. [CrossRef] [PubMed]
18. Clavien, P.A.; Barkun, J.; de Oliveira, M.L.; Vauthey, J.N.; Dindo, D.; Schulick, R.D.; de Santibañes, E.; Pekolj, J.; Slankamenac, K.; Bassi, C.; et al. The Clavien–Dindo classification of surgical complications: Five-year experience. *Ann. Surg.* **2009**, *250*, 187–196. [CrossRef] [PubMed]
19. Dindo, D.; Demartines, N.; Clavien, P.A. Classification of surgical complications: A new proposal with evaluation in a cohort of 6336 patients and results of a survey. *Ann. Surg.* **2004**, *240*, 205–213. [CrossRef] [PubMed]
20. Nagell, J.R., Jr.; Miller, R.W. Evaluation and management of ultrasonographically detected ovarian tumors in asymptomatic women. *Obstet. Gynecol.* **2016**, *127*, 848–858. [CrossRef] [PubMed]
21. National Comprehensive Cancer Network. Epithelial Ovarian Cancer/Fallopian Tube Cancer/Primary Peritoneal Cancer (Version 1.2106). Available online: https://www.nccn.org/professionals/physician_gls/pdf/ovarian.pdf (accessed on 15 November 2016).
22. Goff, B. Symptoms associated with ovarian cancer. *Clin. Obstet. Gynecol.* **2012**, *55*, 36–42. [CrossRef] [PubMed]
23. National Cancer Institute. Surveillance, Epidemiology, and End results Program, Cancer Statistics. Available online: http://seer.cancer.gov/statfacts/ (accessed on 15 November 2016).
24. Alvarado-Cabrero, I.; Navani, S.S.; Young, R.H.; Scully, R.E. Tumors of the fimbriated end of the fallopian tube: A clinicopathologic analysis of 20 cases, including nine carcinomas. *Int. J. Gynecol. Pathol.* **1997**, *16*, 189–196. [CrossRef] [PubMed]
25. Colgan, T.J.; Murphy, J.; Cole, D.E.; Narod, S.; Rosen, B. Occult carcinoma in prophylactic oophorectomy specimens: Prevalence and association with BRCA germline mutation status. *Am. J. Surg. Pathol.* **2001**, *25*, 1283–1289. [CrossRef] [PubMed]
26. Cass, I.; Holschneider, C.; Datta, N.; Barbuto, D.; Walts, A.E.; Karlan, B.Y. BRCA-mutation-associated fallopian tube carcinoma: A distinct clinical phenotype? *Obstet. Gynecol.* **2005**, *106*, 1327–1334. [CrossRef] [PubMed]
27. Medeiros, F.; Muto, M.G.; Lee, Y.; Elvin, J.A.; Callahan, M.J.; Feltmate, C.; Garber, J.E.; Cramer, D.W.; Crum, C.P. The tubal fimbria is a preferred site for early adenocarcinoma in women with familial ovarian cancer syndrome. *Am. J. Surg. Pathol.* **2006**, *30*, 230–236. [CrossRef] [PubMed]
28. Kindelberger, D.W.; Lee, Y.; Miron, A.; Hirsch, M.S.; Feltmate, C.; Medeiros, F.; Callahan, M.J.; Garner, E.O.; Gordon, R.W.; Birch, C.; et al. Intraepithelial carcinoma of the fimbriae and pelvic serous carcinoma: Evidence for a causal relationship. *Am. J. Surg. Pathol.* **2007**, *31*, 161–169. [CrossRef] [PubMed]
29. Crum, C.P.; Drapkin, R.; Miron, A.; Ince, T.A.; Muto, M.; Kindelberger, D.W.; Lee, Y. The distal fallopian tube: A new model for pelvic serous carcinogenesis. *Curr. Opin. Obstet. Gynecol.* **2007**, *19*, 3–9. [CrossRef] [PubMed]
30. Landen, C.N.; Birrer, M.J.; Sood, A.K. Early events in the pathogenesis of epithelial ovarian cancer. *J. Clin. Oncol.* **2008**, *26*, 995–1005. [CrossRef] [PubMed]
31. Lengyel, E. Ovarian cancer development and metastasis. *Am. J. Pathol.* **2010**, *177*, 1053–1064. [CrossRef] [PubMed]
32. Kurman, R.J.; Shih, L.M. The origin and pathogenesis of epithelial ovarian cancer: A proposed unifying theory. *Am. J. Surg. Pathol.* **2010**, *34*, 433–4439. [CrossRef] [PubMed]
33. Crum, C.P.; Mckeon, F.D.; Xian, X. The oviduct and ovarian cancer: Causality, clinical implications, and "Targeted Prevention". *Clin. Obstet. Gynecol.* **2012**, *55*, 24–35. [CrossRef] [PubMed]
34. Cliby, W.A.; Powell, M.A.; Al-Hammadi, N.; Chen, L.; Philip, M.J.; Roland, P.Y.; Mutch, D.G.; Bristow, R.E. Ovarian cancer in the United States: Contemporary patterns of care associated with improved survival. *Gynecol. Oncol.* **2015**, *136*, 11–17. [CrossRef] [PubMed]
35. Bristow, R.E.; Chang, J.; Ziogas, A.; Campos, B.; Chavez, L.R.; Anton-Culver, H. Impact of National Cancer Institute Comprehensive Cancer Centers on ovarian cancer treatment and survival. *J. Am. Coll. Surg.* **2015**, *220*, 940–950. [CrossRef] [PubMed]
36. Bristow, R.E.; Chang, J.; Ziogas, A.; Anton-Culver, H. Adherence to treatment guidelines for ovarian cancer as a measure of quality care. *Obstet. Gynecol.* **2013**, *121*, 1226–1234. [CrossRef] [PubMed]

37. Bristow, R.E.; Palis, B.E.; Chi, D.S.; Cliby, W.A. The National Cancer Database report on advanced-stage epithelial ovarian cancer: Impact of hospital surgical case volume on overall survival and surgical treatment paradigm. *Gynecol. Oncol.* **2010**, *118*, 262–267. [CrossRef] [PubMed]
38. Bristow, R.E.; Chang, J.; Ziogas, A.; Randall, L.M.; Anton-Culver, H. High-volume ovarian cancer care: Survival impact and disparities in access for advanced-stage disease. *Gynecol. Oncol.* **2014**, *132*, 403–410. [CrossRef] [PubMed]
39. Lee, J.Y.; Kim, T.H.; Suh, D.H.; Kim, J.W.; Kim, H.S.; Chung, H.H.; Park, N.H.; Song, Y.S.; Kang, S.B. Impact of guideline adherence on patient outcomes in early-stage epithelial ovarian cancer. *Eur. J. Surg. Oncol.* **2015**, *41*, 585–591. [CrossRef] [PubMed]
40. Vernooij, F.; Heintz, A.P.; Witteveen, P.O.; Coebergh, J.W.; van der Graaf, Y. Specialized care and survival of ovarian cancer patients in The Netherlands: Nationwide cohort study. *J. Natl. Cancer Inst.* **2008**, *100*, 399–406. [CrossRef] [PubMed]

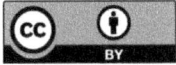

![diagnostics logo] *diagnostics*

MDPI

Article

Symptoms Relevant to Surveillance for Ovarian Cancer

Robert M. Ore [1], Lauren Baldwin [1], Dylan Woolum [1], Erika Elliott [1], Christiaan Wijers [1], Chieh-Yu Chen [1], Rachel W. Miller [1], Christopher P. DeSimone [1], Frederick R. Ueland [1], Richard J. Kryscio [2], John R. van Nagell [1] and Edward J. Pavlik [1,*]

[1] Division of Gynecologic Oncology, Department of Obstetrics and Gynecology, University of Kentucky Chandler Medical Center-Markey Cancer Center, Lexington, KY 40536-0293, USA; robert.ore@uky.edu (R.M.O.); labald1@uky.edu (L.B.); dylan.woolum@uky.edu (D.W.); erikatay28@gmail.com (E.E.); christiaan.d.wijers@vanderbilt.edu (C.W.); chieh-yu.chen@uky.edu (C.-Y.C.); raware00@email.uky.edu (R.W.M.); cpdesi00@uky.edu (C.P.D.); fuela0@email.uky.edu (F.R.U.); jrvann2@email.uky.edu (J.R.v.N.)

[2] Department of Statistics, University of Kentucky Chandler Medical Center-Markey Cancer Center, Lexington, KY 40536-0293, USA; richard.kryscio@uky.edu

* Correspondence: epaul1@uky.edu; Tel.: +1-859-323-3830; Fax: +1-859-323-1018

Academic Editor: Andreas Kjaer
Received: 13 December 2016; Accepted: 13 March 2017; Published: 20 March 2017

Abstract: To examine how frequently and confidently healthy women report symptoms during surveillance for ovarian cancer. A symptoms questionnaire was administered to 24,526 women over multiple visits accounting for 70,734 reports. A query of reported confidence was included as a confidence score (CS). Chi square, McNemars test, ANOVA and multivariate analyses were performed. 17,623 women completed the symptoms questionnaire more than one time and >9500 women completed it more than one four times for >43,000 serially completed questionnaires. Reporting ovarian cancer symptoms was ~245 higher than ovarian cancer incidence. The positive predictive value (0.073%) for identifying ovarian cancer based on symptoms alone would predict one malignancy for 1368 cases taken to surgery due to reported symptoms. Confidence on the first questionnaire (83.3%) decreased to 74% when more than five questionnaires were completed. Age-related decreases in confidence were significant ($p < 0.0001$). Women reporting at least one symptom expressed more confidence (41,984/52,379 = 80.2%) than women reporting no symptoms (11,882/18,355 = 64.7%), $p < 0.0001$. Confidence was unrelated to history of hormone replacement therapy or abnormal ultrasound findings ($p = 0.30$ and 0.89). The frequency of symptoms relevant to ovarian cancer was much higher than the occurrence of ovarian cancer. Approximately 80.1% of women expressed confidence in what they reported.

Keywords: symptoms; questionnaire; certainty/uncertainty

---

1. Introduction

Intake forms are commonly used in clinical care and are often presented to women undergoing well-woman exams and routine gynecologic care. Guidelines exist for British general practitioners [1] as well as for American generalists [2] for collecting and evaluating information on symptoms related to ovarian cancer (OvCA). Women who report certain symptoms are candidates for testing with Ca125, pelvic ultrasound and/or referral to a gynecologic oncologist. Symptoms indicative of ovarian cancer have been included in information collected through the Patient Reported Outcomes Measurement Information System (PROMIS [3,4]) developed by NIH in the United States and integrated with electronic medical records in the ambulatory care setting [5]. Discrepancy has been described between clinician and patient symptoms reporting with many cancer-related symptoms going unrecognized [6]. The dynamics of communication between the physician and patient can be complex and lead to this discrepancy in symptoms discovery with the doctor assuming that the patient will initiate a revealing conversation while the patient expects the doctor to inquire about possible symptoms. Differences in symptoms reporting even exist between paper and electronic reporting [7].

The present report is unique in that it examines factors influencing personal confidence inherent to symptoms reporting by focusing on a large cohort of women without cancer. This report focuses on intake information specific to symptoms of ovarian cancer for deciding the possibility of malignancy. We have employed a questionnaire containing a constellation of symptoms (both related and not related to ovarian cancer) that was reported on by Goff [8]. While data challenging the power of this symptoms index to identify early-stage ovarian cancer has been reported [9,10], symptoms information cannot be ignored, otherwise delays in diagnosis can occur [11]. We have added a self-administered evaluation of reporting confidence to the Goff symptoms questionnaire in order to assess the degree to which women are confident in their responses and have analyzed serially completed questionnaires to determine how time and repeated exposure to symptoms reporting affect confidence. Contemplation of patient-reported confidence is paralleled by the judiciary system where a great deal of emphasis is placed on witness confidence in determining the credibility of testimony [12]. Our report is noteworthy because it identifies changing patient confidence in information that they report on questionnaires which should make physicians more sensitive to the reliability of patient responses.

2. Materials and Methods

Women enrolled in the ongoing ultrasound-based University of Kentucky Ovarian Cancer Screening Program [13–15] from 1987 to July 2013 consisted of both women in the general population and those of high risk based on confirmation of a primary or secondary relative diagnosed with ovarian cancer (n = 41,529). Approval was received from the University of Kentucky Institutional Review Board (IRB number 88-0021-9F6, renewed 11 August 2016). Women were recruited by physician recommendation, media announcements, and word of mouth. Women needed to be competent and understand the terms of the informed consent presented in English, or they were excluded from screening.

Participants in this screening program are characterized as health conscious (>90% medical checkups, >85% annual mammography), well educated (>50% college, ~3% not high school graduates), married (75%) and medically insured (95%) [16].

In October of 2008, participants began completing a modified symptoms questionnaire printed in English which was originally developed by Goff et al. [8]. In total, 24,526 women completed the questionnaire and 17,623 women completed the questionnaire more than once on subsequent screens, for a total of 70,734 evaluated questionnaires. The questionnaire was in the exact form as published by Goff, [8] but was modified to include the confidence of the responder as reported [9]. This modification added the question: "How confidently did you answer these questions?" The possible responses were: "*no confidence*" = 0, "*minimally sure*" = 1, "*more than minimally sure*" = 2, "*pretty sure*" = 3, "*sure*" = 4 and "*absolutely sure*" = 5. The screening sonographer queried each participant about their understanding of each symptom and was responsible for the participant providing answers to all data fields prior to screening. Sonographers gave explanations about the symptoms on the questionnaires as a clarification process prior to screening. Effort was made to model general clinical practice by presenting clarifications as necessary at every participant encounter with the questionnaire. The setting for this study was most similar to women presenting for well-woman exams or routine gynecological checkups. Each questionnaire was completed prior to screening ultrasonography. Over the course of the study 12 different sonographers were involved, each of which received individual training related to questionnaire administration.

Study eligibility, exclusions, instrumentation, protocol, criteria for designating an abnormality, data collection and storage were as previously reported [14,17–19]. In brief, criteria for eligibility were:

(1) women aged $\geq$50 years and (2) women aged 25–49 years with a documented family history of OvCA in at least one primary or secondary relative.

Participants provided their medical history, surgical history, menstrual history/menopausal status, hormonal use, and family history of cancer. Women with a known ovarian tumor or a personal history of OvCA were excluded. Ultrasound findings were designated as abnormal if ovarian volume exceeded 20 cm^3 for pre-menopausal women or 10 cm^3 for post-menopausal women, and if cysts (with septations, solid areas, or papillary projections) as well as echogenic solid structures were observed. An abnormal screening result referred exclusively to the ultrasound result *per se* and not to biomarkers or genetic testing results. Less than 100 women were observed to have free fluid on their ultrasound exam and free fluid generally resolved on their subsequent exam(s) so that free fluid was not treated as an informative predictor.

Following an abnormal ultrasonographic result, repeat screens were scheduled at intervals ranging from six weeks to six months and the symptoms questionnaire was re-administered at each screening. In the present study, the majority of screens were administered annually. The mean interval between questionnaires was 1.15 years $\pm$ 0.01 (SEM), median = 1.03 years, min = 0.02 years/max = 4.9 years, 75th percentile = 1.13 years, 90th percentile = 1.49 years, 95th percentile = 1.95 years. Criteria for *Goff symptoms* related to ovarian cancer were a symptom presenting for >12 days per month with an onset <12 months for having pelvic or abdominal pain, being unable to eat normally, feeling full quickly, feeling abdominal bloating or increased abdominal size. Symptoms *unrelated to ovarian cancer* included on the Goff questionnaire (*non-Goff symptoms*) used in the present study were: back pain, indigestion, nausea, vomiting, weight loss, urinary urgency, frequent urination, constipation, diarrhea, menstrual irregularities, bleeding after menopause, pain during intercourse, fatigue, leg swelling, difficulty breathing.

Confidence of respondents on the symptoms questionnaire was examined in terms of age, menopausal status, body mass index (BMI), hormone replacement therapy (HRT) usage, reporting *no* vs. *any* symptoms, number of Goff symptoms reported, number of non-Goff symptoms reported, number of any symptoms reported and receipt of an abnormal ultrasound screening result. Subjects with missing information listed above were excluded.

Statistical Methods

All information was entered by the sonographer performing the ultrasound into a Medlog database (Medlog Systems, Crystal Bay, NV, USA) using encodings for symptoms, severity, frequency & duration to minimize error on an electronic template organized identically to the printed questionnaire. Random audits of the data and corrections yielded estimates of accuracy greater than 98%. Significance was determined at the $p \leq 0.05$ level in order to robustly identify differences. Proportions were compared using chi-square statistics. In longitudinal analysis, McNemars test for correlated proportions in the marginals was used.

Multivariate analysis: Two binary variables were created from the symptoms confidence scores (CS): (1) *no confidence* defined as a confidence score of 0 versus all other (higher) scores and (2) *little confidence* defined as a score of 0 or 1 versus all other (higher) scores. Each was tabulated against the assessment number. It was decided to abbreviate the assessment number as 1, 2, 3, 4, or 5 plus assessments on the basis of the sample size for each value and due to the fact that the percentage of respondents with no or little confidence did not vary much beyond the fifth time the confidence score was recorded. Similar cross tabulations were done for other potential explanatory variables including BMI (recorded as less than 25, 25–29.99, or 30 plus); presence of HRT (yes or no); number of reported Goff symptoms complying with frequency (>12 days/month) and duration (<12 months) recorded as 0, 1, or 2 plus; abnormal screen (yes or no); menopausal status (premenopausal, postmenopausal, or peri-menopausal); and the number of other symptoms (non-Goff symptoms, recorded as 0, 1–10, and $\geq$11). Age at the assessment was not recoded.

To compare the percentage of "no" or "little" confidence scores among assessments, a generalized linear mixed model was constructed based on a logit link function. Confidence was rated on a six-point Likert (ordinal) scale. The model was fitted using a generalized estimating equation (GEE) procedure to account for repeated assessments on the same subject (working correlation matrix estimated using a compound symmetry assumption). This was done for both a reduced model with only assessment number as a predictor variable and then for a full model with all variables outlined above used as predictor variables. Because the results for the assessment variable were similar for each model, we report only the results for the full model. Statistical significance was determined at the 0.05 level. The GEE models were fitted using PROC GENMOD in PC-SAS, Version 9.3 (SAS Institute, Cary, NC, USA).

3. Results

The demographic characteristics of the group studied are presented in Table 1. None of these women had a diagnosis of ovarian malignancy during the study period or during 40 months of follow-up. Only a small fraction (7.1%) experienced an abnormal ultrasound exam during the study period during which they completed symptoms questionnaires. A total of 24,526 women completed 70,734 symptoms questionnaires (Table 2). The vast majority of participants (prevalence = 88.8%) at some time reported one or more of the constellation of symptoms with only 11.2% never reporting any symptom, shown in Table 2. About a third of reported symptoms (31.9%) occurred on the first questionnaire, while 68.1% had no symptoms on the first reporting. Only 11.5% did not report any symptoms after reporting symptoms on the first report, while about twice as many (20.7%) continued to report symptoms, shown in Table 2. A majority (67.8%) reported symptoms after not having symptoms on the first reporting, accounting for a 60.2% incidence, shown in Table 2. More than 9500 women completed the symptoms questionnaires four or more times, accounting for more than 43,000 symptoms questionnaires completed four or more times (Table 3). Examination of reported confidence on the symptoms questionnaires was made with confidence considered as both a confidence score >0 and >1.

Confidence (CS > 0) was highest on the first questionnaire completed (83.3% of all respondents) and decreased to 74% when five or more questionnaires were completed (Table 4). Complete lack of confidence (CS = 0) in symptoms reporting was observed in 21.1% of all responses and increased (from 16.7% to 26%) as a function of questionnaires completed (Table 4, CS = 0 line), showing decreasing confidence despite increasing experience with the symptoms questionnaire.

Table 1. Demographic characteristics of the study group at first symptom evaluation.

Variable	All, *n* = 24,526 Women
Age	61.7, 61 (24–99)
Parity	2.3, 2 (1–19)
Weight (pounds)	162.4, 156 (76–420)
Height (inches)	64.3, 64 (47–78)
BMI	27.6, 26.6 (12.6–80.5)
Family history of:	
Ovarian cancer	5566 (22.7)
Breast cancer	10,935 (44.6)
Colon cancer	6595 (26.9)
Personal history of:	
Breast cancer	2278 (9.3)
Colon cancer	202 (0.8)
No history of hormone replacement therapy	21,206 (86.5)
History of hormone replacement therapy	3315 (13.5)
Nulliparous	3500 (14.3)
Premenopausal	1597 (6.5)
Perimenopausal	444 (1.8)
Post menopausal	22,840 (93.1)
Abnormal exam history	1742 (7.1)
Any symptoms	18,610 (75.9)
Goff symptoms	845 (3.4)
Other symptoms	16,433 (67.0)

Data are mean, median (range) or *n* (%). BMI: body mass index.

Table 2. Frequency and occurrence of symptoms.

Duration Period of Data Collection Studied 15 April 2008–25 June 2013	
Women screened	24,526 (100%)
Symptoms questionnaires administered	70,734 (100%)
Questionnaires reporting symptoms	52,467 (64.3%)
Women reporting symptoms	21,789 women (88.8%) on 52,467 questionnaires
Women never reporting symptoms	2737 (11.2%)
Women reporting symptoms on first symptoms questionnaire	6956 (31.9% of women reporting symptoms)
Women reporting symptoms with no symptoms on first symptoms questionnaire	14,833 (68.1% of women reporting symptoms)
Women reporting symptoms on first symptoms questionnaire AND subsequently no symptoms reported	2503 (38.2% of women reporting symptoms on 1st questionnaire; 11.5% of all women reporting symptoms)
Women reporting symptoms on first symptoms questionnaire AND subsequently symptoms reported	4515 (68.9% of women reporting symptoms on 1st questionnaire; 20.1% of all women reporting symptoms)
Women reporting NO symptoms on first symptoms questionnaire AND subsequently symptoms	14,771 (99.6% of women with no symptoms on 1st questionnaire; 67.8% of women reporting symptoms)

Table 3. Frequency of symptom questionnaire completion.

Number of Symptoms Questionnaires Completed	Women Completing Questionnaire (*n*)	Total Questionnaires Completed
1	6903	6903
2	4423	8846
3	3696	11,088
4	4530	18,120
5	4168	20,840
6	714	4284
7	84	588
8	7	56
9	1	9
Total	24,526	70,734

Table 4. Confidence as a function of the number of symptoms questionnaires completed.

Confidence	Questionnair Completed	Nunber Completed	Nunber Completed	Nunber Completed	Nunber Completed	Total Completed
Confidence Score (CS)	1st	2nd	3rd	4th	5 or more	All times
0	4103 (16.7)	4055 (23)	2992 (22.7)	2226 (23.4)	1529 (26)	14,905 (21.1)
1	714 (2.9)	443 (2.5)	391 (3)	250 (2.6)	165 (2.8)	1963 (2.8)
2	506 (2.1)	411 (2.3)	349 (2.6)	226 (2.4)	172 (2.9)	1664 (2.4)
3	4090 (16.7)	1984 (11.3)	1353 (10.3)	989 (10.4)	593 (10.1)	9009 (12.7)
4	4280 (17.5)	3477 (19.7)	2774 (21)	2127 (22.4)	1289 (21.9)	13,947 (19.7)
5	10,833 (44.2)	7252 (41.2)	5341 (40.5)	3686 (38.8)	2134 (36.3)	29,246 (41.3)
Responses	24,526 (100)	17,622 (100)	13,200 (100)	9504 (100)	5882 (100)	70,734 (100)
Women completing	1	2	3	4	≥5	Questionnaires
n	6903	4423	3696	4530	4974	24526
Comparisons 1 vs. 2,3,4 or >4	$p < 0.0001$					
2 vs 3, 4		NS $p > 0.5$				
2, 3, 4 vs. >4		$p < 0.0001$				

Response scores were: "no confidence" = 0, "minimally sure" = 1, "more than minimally sure" = 2, "pretty sure" = 3, "sure" = 4 and "absolutely sure" = 5. Analysis for difference included both 0 vs. all other scores and 0 + 1 vs. all other score in both 2×2, 2×6, 2×5 contingency tables. NS: not statistically significant.

3.1. General Factors Associated with Expressions of Confidence in Symptoms Reporting

With increased age, a statistically significant decrease in confidence in symptoms reporting was observed (Table 5), with the fall-off appearing after age 60 so that the ratio of confident to non-confident women over 75 years (2.0) was half that of women under 40 (4.0), shown in Table 5.

Table 5. Confidence as a function of age.

Age, Years	Confidence *n* (%)			Y/N Ratio
	Women	N = No	Y = Yes	
25–40	1073 (1.5)	214 (19.9)	859 (80.1)	4.0
41–50	2911 (4.1)	562 (19.3)	2349 (80.7)	4.2
51–60	21,668 (30.6)	4094 (18.9)	17,574 (81.8)	4.3
61–74	35,900 (50.8)	8972 (25)	26,928 (75)	3.0
≥75	9182 (13)	3026 (33)	6156 (67)	2.0
Total	70,734 (100)	16,868	53,866	

For women under age 40, 80.1% (859/1073) expressed confidence in their response and this decreased to 76.1% for all women over 40 (53,007/69,661), shown in Table 5. Confidence decreased to 75.9% (50,658/66,750) for women over 50, to 73.4% (33,084/45,082) for women over 60 and to 68.9% (11,565/16,778) for women over 70 ($p < 0.0001$). Expressed confidence for postmenopausal women was 75.7% (49,100/64,831), mirroring confidence for women over 50 years of age.

The fraction of underweight (BMI ≤ 18.5) and normal weight (BMI = 18.5–24.9) women who expressed confidence in their reporting (21,263/27,932 = 76.1%) was not significantly different from overweight (BMI = 25–29.9) and obese (BMI ≥ 30) responders (32,603/42,802 = 76.2%). The fraction of women that received an abnormal screening result and expressed confidence in their reporting only differed by 1% from the fraction of women that had a normal screening result, while for only Goff symptoms the difference was 6% and not statistically significant.

Significantly more women reporting at least one symptom expressed confidence in their responses (41,984/52,379 = 80.2%) than women who reported no symptoms (11,882/18,355 = 64.7%), $p < 0.0001$. Women that reported at least one Goff symptom relevant to ovarian cancer expressed confidence with the same frequency (1597/1931 = 82.7%) as women that did not report any Goff symptoms (9895/11,871 = 83.4%). There were more women that expressed confidence who reported at least one of the symptoms (those not relevant to ovarian cancer) (37,163/45,992 = 80.8%) than women who did not report any symptoms (16,703/24,742 = 67.5%), $p < 0.0001$. Thus, participants that were the least certain about what they reported were those women who did not report having symptoms.

3.2. Longitudinal Analysis of Confidence Stability

Efforts were directed at determining if confidence scores changed as individuals completed more symptoms evaluations. Analysis focused on 17,623 individuals who completed two or more symptoms questionnaires. Results were based on individuals initially reporting some confidence (CS > 0) and tracked on the basis of the number of symptoms questionnaires that were completed. The change between the first and last confidence score was determined for each individual as increasing, decreasing or unchanged. The fraction of women that demonstrated a decrease in confidence expanded as additional questionnaires were completed (Figure 1). Confidence remained unchanged in approximately one-third of the cases (35.1%–37.4%, Table 6). Confidence scores increased in ~20% of women that initially reported some confidence (CS > 0: 18.4%–22.6%, Table 6). Decreases in confidence occurred in just under 50% of the individuals that initially reported some confidence (CS > 0: 41.4%–46%, Table 6). There was a statistically significant difference in the response distribution between individuals completing the questionnaire two to three times vs. those taking the questionnaire five or more times ($p < 0.005$), shown in Table 6. Examining paired longitudinal differences using the McNemars test showed a significant difference ($p < 0.0001$) for completing three, four, or five or more evaluations compared to two evaluations (Table 6). Thus, longitudinal analysis indicated a trending decrease of confidence scores (Table 6) in almost half of the women completing the symptoms questionnaires.

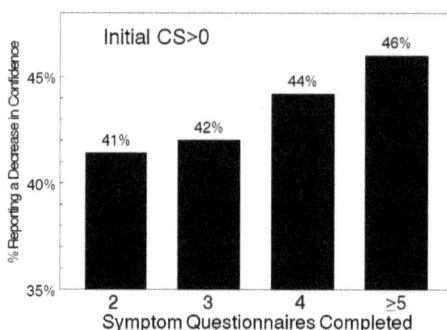

Figure 1. Confidence reported as a function of the number of symptoms questionnaires completed. Decreased confidence reported by women who originally reported confidence (CS > 0).

Table 6. Longitudinal stability as a function of the number of symptoms questionnaires completed (CS > 0).

Questionnaires Completed	Change	*n*	%	Comparison	Significance
2	a. Increased	827	22.6%	2 vs. 3, 4	NS
2	b. Unchanged	1318	36.0%	2 vs. ≥5	$p < 0.005$
2	c. Decreased	1518	41.4%		
2	Sub-total	3663	100.0%		
3	a. Increased	688	22.3%	3 vs. 4	NS
3	b. Unchanged	1101	35.7%	3 vs. ≥5	$p < 0.005$
3	c. Decreased	1297	42.0%		
3	Sub-total	3086	100.0%		
4	a. Increased	708	18.4%	4 vs. ≥5	NS
4	b. Unchanged	1439	37.4%		
4	c. Decreased	1702	44.2%		
4	Sub-total	3849	100.0%		
≥5	a. Increased	793	18.8%	4 vs. ≥5	NS
≥5	b. Unchanged	1478	35.1%	3 vs. ≥5	$p < 0.005$
≥5	c. Decreased	1936	46.0%	2 vs. ≥5	$p < 0.005$
≥5	Sub-total	4207	100.0%		

Significance in the table is based on chi square 3 × 2 contingency table analyses. $p < 0.0001$ using McNemars test for correlated proportions in the marginals of a 2 × 2 contingency table for initial confidence >0 where decreased paired confidence = "Yes". Comparisons were for two to five or more evaluations. Odds ratio changed from 1.18 (two vs. three evaluations) to 1.496 (two vs. five or more evaluations). $p < 0.0001$ using McNemars test for initial confidence = 0 where increased confidence = "Yes".

3.3. Multivariate Analysis

Relating the binary outcome (confidence scale) to the number of symptoms questionnaires completed was based on the frequencies reported in column 2 of Table 3 and not on arbitrarily varying the cut point to achieve significant results. The percentage of respondents expressing no confidence increased significantly from 16.7% after the first assessment ($p < 0.0001$ when each of the no confidence levels for assessments two, three, four, or five plus were compared to the first assessment). It then leveled off during assessments two, three, or four (23.0%, 22.7%, and 23.4%, respectively) which were not statistically different from each other. However, by assessment five or later, those expressing no confidence increased to 26.0% which is significant when compared to assessments two, three, or four ($p < 0.001$ in all cases). All other variables examined were significant in the multivariate model except for use of hormone replacement therapy ($p = 0.44$), and normal vs. abnormal screening exams ($p = 0.09$). Thus, although the number of women with abnormal findings is small, so it should be expected to have little effect in this study, it does not test as a confounder. Specifically, the percentage of patients expressing no confidence increased with age ($p < 0.001$). The percentage was stable through age 60 and then increased steadily from 18.8% to 32.8% by age 85; decreased for morbidly obese patients (19.9% compared to normal BMI 21.2%, ($p < 0.03$); declined with the number of other symptoms reported (symptoms unrelated to ovarian cancer) from 31.2% (score 0) to 18.5% (scores 1 through 10) to 6.4% (score 11); decreased with the number of reported Goff symptoms complying with frequency (>12 days/month) and duration (<12 months) from 21.3% at score 0 to 15.1% at score 1 to 12.1% for scores ≥ 2; and increased in postmenopausal women when compared to premenopausal women (21.3% versus 19.3%, $p < 0.0001$). Similar results were obtained for the endpoint *little confidence* (results not shown).

3.4. Symptoms Reported Relevant to Ovarian Cancer

Overall, 59.9% (42,404/70,734) of the symptoms questionnaires reported one or more of the five symptoms related to ovarian cancer, but only 3.9% (2756/70,734) met the frequency and duration criteria and did so with a significantly different distribution (Table 7. $p < 0.0001$). The overall incidence of symptoms was: abdominal bloating > pelvic pain > increased abdominal size > feeling full quickly > unable to eat normally (Table 7). In these women that were not diagnosed with an ovarian malignancy during the study period or during 40 months of follow-up, the incidence of any of the five symptoms relevant to ovarian cancer was high, but frequency and duration information significantly reduced this number. Symptom severity was significantly lower in women that did not meet the Goff-positive frequency and duration criteria ($p < 0.001$, Table 7), but did not differ with regards to reported confidence (CS = 0 vs. CS > 0). Most women (68.4%, Table 8) reported only one symptom that met the Goff criteria of frequency and duration, while 23.3% reported two and ~8% reported three or more of these symptoms (Table 8). Moreover, the incidence of symptoms was not different with respect to reported confidence (CS = 0 vs. CS > 0). Nevertheless, the 2.7% Goff-positive occurrence (Table 8: 1931/70,734) was nearly ~245 times higher than the ovarian cancer incidence for this population (11.2/100,000), [20]. Unlike one-time reports that have previously considered symptoms related to ovarian cancer, the present report is a longitudinal study of multiple reports collected over time. Consequently, a woman may be positive for the Goff ovarian cancer symptoms in the context of always meeting or sometimes meeting the frequency and duration criteria. There are also women in the present data set who, after being positive for the Goff ovarian cancer symptoms, subsequently no longer report these symptoms. Against this background, to address these considerations, we identify two groups: (A) women that at any time have reported any Goff ovarian cancer symptoms and (B) women that at any time satisfied the frequency and duration criteria for any Goff ovarian cancer symptoms. Approximately one-third of the women surveyed (7983/24,526) qualified for inclusion in Group A, while ~7% of women qualified for inclusion in Group B (1708/24,526). Our estimates mirror a recent report from the United Kingdom on ovarian cancer symptoms reported in the general population [21]. In relating these findings to the positive predictive value (PPV) which depends on prevalence (PPV = True Positives/(True Positives + False Positives)), the work presented here would yield a symptoms-estimated PPV of 0.073% or one malignancy for 1368 cases that would be taken to surgery using the sample reported on here (24,526 women filling out 70,734 questionnaires reporting 52,467 symptoms for 21,789 women) and screen-detected ovarian cancers reported previously [9]. This symptoms-estimated PPV is smaller than that reported by Rossing from a much smaller study size ($n = 1905$) [10] that would not have approached prevalence as closely as the results described here. However, despite the occurrence of symptoms being vastly higher than the incidence of ovarian cancer, ignoring symptoms is very likely to result in women being diagnosed with advanced-stage disease [11].

Table 7. Occurrence of symptoms related to ovarian cancer.

Symptom	Goff-Negative Occurrence Freq < 12 per Month and Duration > 12 Months, *n* (%)	CS = 0	Severity	CS > 0	Severity
Pelvic Pain	10,859 (25.6)	1702 (24.3)	2.1 ± 0.03	9157 (25.9)	2.1 ± 0.01
Unable to eat normally	2584 (6.1)	459 (6.6)	2.2 ± 0.06	2125 (6)	2.2 ± 0.03
Feeling full quickly	5566 (13.1)	960 (13.7)	2.2 ± 0.04	4606 (13)	2.1 ± 0.02
Abdominal bloating	14,934 (35.2)	2477 (35.4)	2.2 ± 0.02	12,457 (35.2)	2.2 ± 0.01
Increased abdominal size	8461 (20)	1396 (20)	2.3 ± 0.03	7065 (20)	2.3 ± 0.02
Total	42404 (100)	6994 (100)		35,410 (100)	
Symptom	Goff-Positive Occurrence Freq > 12 per Month and Duration < 12 Months, *n* (%)	CS = 0	Severity	CS > 0	Severity
Pelvic Pain	588 (21.3)	86 (22.6)	3.1 ± 0.13	502 (21.1)	3.04 ± 0.05
Unable to eat normally	244 (8.9)	36 (9.5)	3.1 ± 0.21	208 (8.8)	3.5 ± 0.09
Feeling full quickly	446 (16.2)	62 (16.3)	3.3 ± 0.15	384 (16.2)	3.2 ± 0.06
Abdominal bloating	832 (30.2)	115 (30.2)	3.5 ± 0.1	717 (30.2)	3.4 ± 0.04
Increased abdominal size	646 (23.4)	82 (21.5)	3.4 ± 0.13	564 (23.8)	3.12 ± 0.05
Total	2756 (100)	381 (100)		2375 (100)	

Severity was reported using the scale: 1 = minimal to 5 = severe (mean ± SEM). Severity Goff-negative vs. Goff-positive: $p < 0.001$.

Table 8. Occurrence of multiple symptoms.

Number of Symptoms	Goff-Positive Occurrence Freq > 12 per Month and Duration < 12 Months, *n* (%)	CS = 0	CS > 0
1	1321 (68.4)	200 (73)	1121 (67.7)
2	450 (23.3)	49 (17.9)	401 (24.2)
3	115 (6)	18 (6.6)	97 (5.9)
4	35 (1.8)	6 (2.2)	29 (1.8)
5	10 (0.5)	1 (0.4)	9 (0.5)
Total	1931 (100)	274 (100)	1657 (100)

CS = 0 vs. CS > 0: $p = 0.23$.

4. Discussion

This is the first work to examine symptoms related to ovarian cancer in a very large sample and to consider the confidence that women, all with an eventual non-surgical outcome, have in the responses they entered on a symptoms questionnaire that they completed prior to their ultrasound exam. A significant finding of the work presented here is that a large majority of women (80.1%) were confident in their reporting. Confidence was lowest (64.7%) in women who did not report any symptoms. Decreasing confidence despite increasing experience with the questionnaire was demonstrated by the finding that the fraction lacking confidence increased as a function of the number of times that the symptoms questionnaire was completed. Importantly, confidence scores in individuals followed longitudinally showed a decreasing trend in almost 50% of women. There was a significant age-related decrease in confidence, and women that did not report any symptoms were significantly less confident than women who reported at least one symptom. Importantly, confidence decreased as more symptoms were reported, including both ovarian cancer–related Goff symptoms complying with frequency (>12 days/month) and duration (<12 months), as well as other symptoms unrelated to ovarian cancer. Thus, reporting of an increased number of symptoms did not coincide with greater confidence in the results reported. Analyses of symptom severity indicated that severity was higher in women that met the Goff-positive frequency and duration criteria than in women that did not, suggesting that transient or long-standing symptoms may be of lower intensity. It is noteworthy that symptoms reporting was done prior to receiving an ultrasound exam with the result that there was no statistically significant difference in confidence between women receiving a normal vs. abnormal sonographic result.

These findings indicate that while *uncertainty in symptoms reporting* occurs to a much lesser extent than certainty, every individual's report must be carefully assessed and not unconditionally accepted. It may even be appropriate to consider serial evaluation of symptoms in order for physicians to understand the extent to which complaints continue to persist or resolve. The symptoms questionnaire utilized here includes reporting of frequency and duration in addition to the actual symptoms. Consequently, uncertainty about frequency and duration may be contributing to how an individual's response reflects confidence in what they report on the questionnaire. Memory certainly plays a role in recalling when symptoms began and how often they have occurred, and this may become more challenging as a person gets older. Thus, age-related effects on memory may be most relevant to certainty about the frequency and duration of symptoms and, with multiple co-morbidities that accumulate over time, can make it difficult to identify a "new" symptom per se or to pinpoint its onset. It is also possible that as a person gets older, they become accepting of many of the symptoms considered here occurring sporadically or episodically and as such are reluctant to declare them a symptom of anything other than age.

An impact on the healthcare delivery system arises when symptoms related to ovarian cancer are reported by women that do not have an ovarian malignancy and can result in inappropriate clinical decisions that could lead to unnecessary surgery. Some data exist supporting symptoms-based surveillance with even early cancers producing symptoms detectable by questionnaire [22]. Symptoms reporting is currently important for the identification of patients needing imaging and closer examination. Just as a lack of witness confidence in legal testimony raises questions about credibility, physicians should be sensitive to the same possibility being relevant to over-diagnosis and over-treatment if a patient may be uncertain about what they report. In addition, certainty about symptoms should not be mistaken to be related to the presence of pathology. Physicians should be made aware that confidence will decrease with age and that reporting multiple symptoms does not imply patient confidence or credibility in the report. Thus, physicians should deliberate through patient information in order to make appropriate assignments of diagnostic tests and follow-up.

The strengths of this study include the large number of patients participating, and the large number of patients completing questionnaires on more than one occasion. In addition, trained sonographers assisted participants in collecting their medical history by answering questions about the context of the questionnaires that participants were filling out. The present report focuses on the level of confidence women have in reporting symptoms as a statistical estimation and not hypothesis testing. It investigates factors that might alter this level and while this involves hypothesis testing, the large sample size assures adequate statistical power to identify some factors that do affect the reported confidence level.

The inherent weakness of a study of this nature is its subjective nature. One person's symptom may be something that someone else has become accustomed to. Subjectivity also occurred in the confidence scale; however, its gradation allowed different dichotomization points to be examined to delineate certainty from uncertainty. It is also possible that a lack of confidence associated with reporting an increased number of symptoms reflects a lack of confidence in only part of the symptoms reported on the questionnaire but not in others. This possibility was not examined in the design that was utilized because addressing this would add the burden of 63 individual confidence assessments (i.e., confidence assessments for 21 symptoms, amplified by confidence queries on severity, frequency and duration: $21 \times 3 = 63$). Understanding the context of the questionnaire certainly has an influence on confidence. The questionnaire used here included reporting of severity, frequency and duration in addition to the symptoms per se. Consequently, uncertainty about severity, frequency and duration may contribute to how an individual response reflects confidence.

Directions for future study might include an assessment of whether the levels of confidence reported here are chiefly related to completing a printed questionnaire and how they also extend to interviews with healthcare professionals. The discrepancy between clinician and patient symptoms ratings is greatest for more subjective symptoms [23]. To this end, it must be realized that clinician symptom ratings are lower than patient-reported ratings [24,25]. Consequently, care must be taken about assuming the superiority of information on symptoms gathered by clinicians and about the inferiority of patient-reported symptoms. Likewise, the results here indicate that uncertainty can exist in patient-reported symptoms.

5. Clinical Implications

Although the balance between patient confidence and uncertainty very heavily favors confidence, the level of *uncertainty in symptoms reporting* described here should be kept in mind when extracting symptoms information from patients. This principle may affect the extent to which symptoms information is relied upon or should be probed during the clinical evaluation process. The addition of psychosocial tools to evaluate the contributions of stress, anxiety and depression need to be explored to help the clinician extract the pertinent information from patient symptoms reporting so that those most at risk for malignancy can be identified.

Acknowledgments: This work will be submitted in partial fulfillment of the required thesis of Robert M. Ore for his Fellowship in Gynecologic Oncology. This work was supported by grants from the Telford Foundation, and the Department of Health and Human Services, Commonwealth of Kentucky.

Author Contributions: Robert M. Ore contributed to data summary review, abstract composition and manuscript construction; Lauren Baldwin contributed to concept development and manuscript organization; Dylan Woolum, Erika Elliott, and Christiaan Wijers contributed to data collection and review. Chieh-Yu Chen contributed to Python programming for data isolation; Rachel W. Miller, Christopher P. DeSimone, and Frederick R. Ueland contributed to manuscript preparation. Richard J. Kryscio performed statistical analysis and contributed to manuscript preparation. John R. van Nagell, contributed to manuscript preparation. Edward J. Pavlik developed the project concept, organized the data collection methdlogy, and contributed to data quality control, symptoms reporting integrity, statistical evaluation and manuscript composition. The authors are solely responsible for subject development, data collection & analysis, and composition.

Conflicts of Interest: The authors declare that there are no conflicts of interest.

References

1. National Institute for Health and Clinical Excellence. Ovarian Cancer: The Recognition and Initial Management of Ovarian Cancer. Clinical Guidelines CG122. Edited by NICE. April 2011, Volume CG122. Available online: http://www.nice.org.uk/guidance/cg122 (accessed on 22 February 2017).
2. ACOG Committee Opinion No. 280: The role of the generalist obstetrician-gynecologist in the early detection of ovarian cancer. *Obstet. Gynecol.* **2002**, *100*, 1413–1416.
3. Cella, D.; Riley, W.; Stone, A.; Rothrock, N.; Reeve, B.; Yount, S.; Amtmann, D.; Bode, R.; Buysse, D.; Choi, S.; et al. The Patient-Reported Outcomes Measurement Information System (PROMIS) developed and tested its first wave of adult self-reported health outcome item banks: 2005–2008. *J. Clin. Epidemiol.* **2010**, *63*, 1179–1194. [CrossRef] [PubMed]
4. Pilkonis, P.A.; Choi, S.W.; Reise, S.P.; Stover, A.M.; Riley, W.T.; Cella, D. Item banks for measuring emotional distress from the Patient-Reported Outcomes Measurement Information System (PROMIS): Depression, anxiety, and anger. *Assessment* **2011**, *18*, 263–283. [CrossRef] [PubMed]
5. Wagner, L.I.; Schink, J.; Bass, M.; Patel, S.; Diaz, M.V.; Rothrock, N.; Pearman, T.; Gershon, R.; Penedo, F.J.; Rosen, S.; et al. Bringing PROMIS to practice: Brief and precise symptom screening in ambulatory cancer care. *Cancer* **2015**, *121*, 927–934. [CrossRef] [PubMed]
6. Vogelzang, N.J.; Breitbart, W.; Cella, D.; Curt, G.A.; Groopman, J.E.; Horning, S.J.; Itri, L.M.; Johnson, D.H.; Scherr, S.L.; Portenoy, R.K. Patient, caregiver, and oncologist perceptions of cancer-related fatigue: Results of a tripart assessment survey. The Fatigue Coalition. *Semin. Hematol.* **1997**, *34*, 4–12. [PubMed]
7. Dupont, A.; Wheeler, J.; Herndon, I.J.E.; Coan, A.; Zafar, S.Y.; Hood, L.; Patwardhan, M.; Shaw, H.S.; Lyerly, H.K.; Abernethy, A.P. Use of tablet personal computers for sensitive patient-reported information. *J. Support. Oncol.* **2009**, *7*, 91–97. [PubMed]
8. Goff, B.A.; Mandel, L.S.; Drescher, C.W.; Urban, N.; Gough, S.; Schurman, K.M.; Patras, J.; Mahony, B.S.; Andersen, M.R. Development of an ovarian cancer symptom Index: Possibilities for earlier detection. *Cancer* **2007**, *109*, 221–227. [CrossRef] [PubMed]

9. Pavlik, E.J.; Saunders, B.A.; Doran, S.; McHugh, K.W.; Ueland, F.R.; DeSimone, C.P.; Depriest, P.D.; Ware, R.A.; Kryscio, R.J.; van Nagell, J.R., Jr. The search for meaning—Symptoms and transvaginal sonography screening for ovarian cancer. *Cancer* **2009**, *115*, 3689–3698. [CrossRef] [PubMed]
10. Rossing, M.A.; Wicklund, K.G.; Cushing-Haugen, K.L.; Weiss, N.S. Predictive value of symptoms for early detection of ovarian cancer. *J. Natl. Cancer Inst.* **2010**, *102*, 222–229. [CrossRef] [PubMed]
11. Goff, B. Symptoms associated with ovarian cancer. *Clin. Obstet. Gynecol.* **2012**, *55*, 36–42. [CrossRef] [PubMed]
12. Bornstein, B.H.; Zickafoose, D.J. "I know I know it, I know I saw it": The stability of the confidence-accuracy relationship across domains. *J. Exp. Psychol.* **1999**, *5*, 76–88. [CrossRef]
13. Higgins, R.; Nagell, J.R.; Donaldson, E.S.; Gallion, H.H.; Pavlik, E.J.; Endicott, B.; Woods, C.H. Transvaginal sonography as a screening method for ovarian cancer. *Gynecol. Oncol.* **1989**, *34*, 402–406. [CrossRef]
14. DePriest, P.D.; Gallion, H.H.; Pavilk, E.J.; Kryscio, R.K.; van Nagell, J.R. Transvaginal sonography as a screening method for the detection of early ovarian cancer. *Gynecol. Oncol.* **1997**, *65*, 408–414. [CrossRef] [PubMed]
15. Van Nagell, J.R.; Pavlik, E.J. Ovarian cancer screening. *Clin. Obstet. Gynecol.* **2012**, *55*, 43–51. [CrossRef] [PubMed]
16. Pavlik, E.J.; Johnson, T.L.; DePriest, P.D.; Andrykowski, M.A.; Kryscio, R.J.; Nagell, J.R.; van Nagell, J.R., Jr. Continuing participation supports ultrasound screening for ovarian cancer. *Ultrasound Obstet. Gynecol.* **2000**, *15*, 354–364. [CrossRef] [PubMed]
17. Ueland, F.R.; DePriest, P.; DeSimone, C.; Pavlik, E.J.; Lele, S.M.; Kryscio, R.J.; van Nagell, J.R., Jr. The accuracy of examination under anesthesia and transvaginal sonography in evaluating ovarian size. *Gynecol. Oncol.* **2005**, *99*, 400–403. [CrossRef] [PubMed]
18. Pavlik, E.J.; DePriest, P.D.; Gallion, H.H.; Ueland, F.R.; Reedy, M.B.; Kryscio, R.J.; van Nagell, J.R., Jr. Ovarian volume related to age. *Gynecol. Oncol.* **2000**, *77*, 410–412. [CrossRef] [PubMed]
19. Van Nagell, J.R.; DePriest, P.; Reedy, M.; Gallion, H.H.; Ueland, F.R.; Pavlik, E.J.; Kryscio, R.J. The efficacy of transvaginal sonographic screening in asymptomatic women at risk for ovarian cancer. *Gynecol. Oncol.* **2000**, *77*, 350–356. [CrossRef] [PubMed]
20. U.S. Cancer Statistics Working Group. United States Cancer Statistics: 1999–2013 Incidence and Mortality Web-based Report. Atlanta: U.S. Department of Health and Human Services, Centers for Disease Control and Prevention and National Cancer Institute, 2016. Available online: www.cdc.gov/uscs (accessed on 22 February 2017).
21. Lim, A.W.; Mesher, D.; Sasieni, P. Estimating the workload associated with symptoms-based ovarian cancer screening in primary care: An audit of electronic medical records. *BMC Fam. Pract.* **2014**, *15*, 1–6. [CrossRef] [PubMed]
22. Goff, B.A.; Mandel, L.; Muntz, H.G.; Melancon, C.H. Ovarian carcinoma diagnosis. *Cancer* **2000**, *89*, 2068–2075. [CrossRef]
23. Basch, E.; Iasonos, A.; McDonough, T.; Barz, A.; Culkin, A.; Kris, M.G.; Scher, H.I.; Schrag, D. Patient versus clinician symptom reporting using the National Cancer Institute Common Terminology Criteria for Adverse Events: Results of a questionnaire-based study. *Lancet Oncol.* **2006**, *7*, 903–909. [CrossRef]
24. Basch, E. The missing voice of patients in drug-safety reporting. *N. Engl. J. Med.* **2010**, *362*, 865–869. [CrossRef] [PubMed]
25. Fromme, E.K.; Eilers, K.M.; Mori, M.; Hsieh, Y.C.; Beer, T.M. How accurate is clinician reporting of chemotherapy adverse effects? A comparison with patient-reported symptoms from the Quality-of-Life Questionnaire C30. *J. Clin. Oncol.* **2004**, *22*, 3485–3490. [CrossRef] [PubMed]

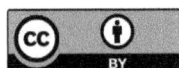

diagnostics

MDPI

Article

Ovarian Cancer Incidence Corrected for Oophorectomy

Lauren A. Baldwin [1,*], Quan Chen [2], Thomas C. Tucker [3], Connie G. White [4], Robert N. Ore [1] and Bin Huang [2]

[1] The Division of Gynecologic Oncology, Department of Obstetrics and Gynecology, The University of Kentucky College of Medicine, 800 Rose Street, 330 Whitney-Hendrickson Building, Lexington, KY 40536, USA; robert.ore@uky.edu

[2] Division of Cancer Biostatistics, College of Public Health & Biostatistics Shared Resource Facility, Markey Cancer Center, University of Kentucky, Lexington, KY 40506, USA; quan.chen@uky.edu (Q.C.); bhuang@kcr.uky.edu (B.H.)

[3] Department of Epidemiology, College of Public Health & Kentucky Cancer Registry, Markey Cancer Center, University of Kentucky, Lexington, KY 40506, USA; tct@kcr.uky.edu

[4] Kentucky Department for Public Health, Frankfort, KY 40601, USA; Connie.White@ky.gov

* Correspondence: labald1@uky.edu; Tel.: +1-859-323-9880; Fax: +1-859-323-1602

Academic Editor: Tanya W. Moseley
Received: 30 December 2016; Accepted: 18 March 2017; Published: 1 April 2017

Abstract: Current reported incidence rates for ovarian cancer may significantly underestimate the true rate because of the inclusion of women in the calculations who are not at risk for ovarian cancer due to prior benign salpingo-oophorectomy (SO). We have considered prior SO to more realistically estimate risk for ovarian cancer. Kentucky Health Claims Data, International Classification of Disease 9 (ICD-9) codes, Current Procedure Terminology (CPT) codes, and Kentucky Behavioral Risk Factor Surveillance System (BRFSS) Data were used to identify women who have undergone SO in Kentucky, and these women were removed from the at-risk pool in order to re-assess incidence rates to more accurately represent ovarian cancer risk. The protective effect of SO on the population was determined on an annual basis for ages 5–80+ using data from the years 2009–2013. The corrected age-adjusted rates of ovarian cancer that considered SO ranged from 33% to 67% higher than age-adjusted rates from the standard population. Correction of incidence rates for ovarian cancer by accounting for women with prior SO gives a better understanding of risk for this disease faced by women. The rates of ovarian cancer were substantially higher when SO was taken into consideration than estimates from the standard population.

Keywords: ovarian cancer; prevalence; incidence; oophorectomy; screening

1. Introduction

Cancer incidence rates are calculated by dividing new primary cancer cases of a disease by the population at risk in the same time period adjusted by the US standard population [1]. This assessment has great importance clinically, especially for gynecologic oncology with regard to training a sufficient number of physician specialists. Cancer incidence rates help physicians and researchers assess risk levels, which can be used for public health and individual patient education, to prioritize prevention and research efforts, and to guide assessment of the cost and efficacy of cancer screening. Thus, the accuracy of this risk assessment is very important.

There is an inherent problem in the incidence calculation for some malignancies due to the inclusion of patients in the denominator who are not at risk for the disease [2]. In gynecologic oncology, this has been most thoroughly evaluated in the case of endometrial cancer and hysterectomy. Many women will undergo hysterectomy in their lifetime for a variety of benign conditions [3,4]. These women are not at risk for developing endometrial cancer after uterine removal and should not be included in the population at risk for incidence rate calculation. There have been multiple publications that have evaluated methods of correcting risk calculations for endometrial cancer. In 2012, Siegel et al. reported on age-adjusted, hysterectomy-corrected uterine cancer rates stratified by race and geography and found that failure to adjust rates for hysterectomy leads to distortion of racial and geographic patterns and underestimates disease burden [5].

There is less guidance in the literature concerning the impact of oophorectomy rates on ovarian cancer incidence. Many women have salpingo-oophorectomy (SO) performed alone due to benign ovarian disease, or have SO performed at the time of hysterectomy for benign conditions. There has been new evidence linking the origin of serous ovarian cancer to the fimbriated end of the fallopian tube [6–17]. During adnexal surgeries, the tube is usually removed concurrently with the ovary. Whether the pathogenesis for the most common type of ovarian cancer truly arises from the distal tube or the ovary itself, those who have undergone SO should have drastically reduced risk of this type of malignancy. This reduction has been demonstrated in high risk women with Breast Cancer Susceptibility (*BRCA*) mutations who undergo risk-reducing salpingo-oophorectomy and have dramatically lower risk of ovarian malignancy [16–19].

The current reported incidence of ovarian cancer from 2005–2009 is 12.7 per 100,000 women [20]. Incidence rates are higher in whites and the average age at diagnosis is 63 [20]. Lifetime risk of developing ovarian cancer in the United States is 1.4% [20]. In 2016, 22,280 new cases were expected and 14,240 deaths anticipated from this disease [21]. Ovarian cancer is the 5th leading cause of death from malignancy in women in this country due to the fact that the majority of cases are diagnosed at an advanced stage. Research into prevention and screening for ovarian cancer is hampered by this low prevalence, which negatively affects accurately estimating the positive predictive value for these tests. We hypothesize that when incidence rates are corrected for prior SO, incidence of this disease will be higher than in commonly reported statistics which currently underestimate the risk of ovarian cancer for women whose ovaries and/or tubes remain intact.

2. Materials and Methods

2.1. Cancer Incidence Data

To calculate the cancer incidence rates, the most recent five-year ovary cancer cases diagnosed in years 2009–2013 from the Kentucky Cancer Registry (KCR) were extracted. Ovary cancer cases were defined as ICD-O-3 site codes C569 excluding ICD-O-3 histology codes 9050–9055, 9140, 9590–9992. Only invasive cancer cases were included for the analysis.

The KCR is a population-based registry, and has been awarded the highest level of certification by the North American Association of Central Cancer Registries for an objective evaluation of completeness, accuracy, and timeliness every year since 1997. The KCR is part of both the CDC National Program of Cancer Registries and the NCI Surveillance, Epidemiology, and End Results (SEER) program, which are considered among the most accurate and complete population-based cancer registries in the world. The KCR also links its database annually with the National Death Index (NDI) to capture the most accurate survival information. No new data was collected from subjects specifically for this study and no contact with any patients was required. All data was previously de-identified.

2.2. Kentucky Health Claims Data (KHCD)

In order to correctly calculate the age-adjusted rates for ovary cancer incidence, the underlying risk population needs to be modified to reflect the fact that women who had SO will have minimal risk of having ovarian cancer. To estimate the prevalence of women who had prior SO for years 2009–2013 in Kentucky, the Kentucky health claims data (KHCD) 2000–2014 data sets were acquired from the Office of Health Policy in the Kentucky Cabinet for Health and Family Services (KCHFS).

The KHCD data include hospital discharge reports from all Kentucky hospitals, Medicare provider-based entities and ambulatory facilities (http://lrc.ky.gov/KAR/900/007/030.htm). The data include in-patient and out-patient files containing de-identified individual records. Key elements, such as ICD-9 procedure codes, CPT codes, and demographics are included in the files. Age is presented in the format of age groups.

2.3. Kentucky Behavioral Risk Factor Surveillance System (BRFSS) Data

The Behavioral Risk Factor Surveillance System (BRFSS) data is the annual telephone survey that collects state data related to health risk behavior, chronic health conditions, and use of preventive services for all 50 states, the District of Columbia, and three territories in the U.S (https://www.cdc.gov/brfss/). For women aged 18 and older, responses to the question "Have you had a hysterectomy?" are included. The data related to this question was used to estimate the prevalence of prior hysterectomy by age group. Since the hysterectomy question was presented every other year, the Kentucky BRFSS data 2008–2012 was acquired from the KCHFS to match the ovary cancer incidence data 2009–2013.

2.4. Estimating Oophorectomy Prevalence

To estimate the prevalence of prior SO for Kentucky women in 2009–2013, two approaches were used. The first method estimated the full SO prevalence rates directly from the KHCD data and the second method estimated the SO prevalence rates based on both BRFSS data and KHCD data.

In the first method, SO cases were identified by ICD-9 procedure codes and CPT codes from the KHCD data for the years 2000–2014. Since the KHCD data in 2000–2003 did not include age or CPT codes and 2014 data were beyond the study period, only data for years 2004–2013 were used for the data analysis. The combined counts of SO cases by year and age group from both in-patient and out-patient files were considered as the total SO incidence. The age groups in KHCD data were categorized as 0, 1–5, 6–10, ... , 76–80, 81+ years. Statistical approaches to estimating prevalence from incidence data commonly involves mortality and survival data, and can be either parametric or non-parametric [22–25]. Counting Method, a non-parametric approach, was used to estimate prevalence of prior SO based on the SO incidence data from the KHCD [23]. This approach counts cases of 'still alive' individuals on the desired prevalence date while making adjustment based on the estimates of cases lost to follow-up. For example, the number of prevalence case in age i and calendar year j was estimated as

$$N_{ij} = \int_0^i I(t)S(t, i - t)dt$$

where $I(t)$ is the number of incidence in age t, and $S(t, i - t)$ is the survival probability from all causes from age t to $i - t$. Since the KHCD data do not include survival and mortality data, the US 2010 female life tables were used to estimate the survival probabilities from all causes in the specific years and age groups. Bridged life tables to match the age group defined in the KHCD were calculated from the complete US 2010 female life table [26]. Because no SO incidence data by age group were available prior to 2004, it was assumed that the incidence data prior to 2004 were same as in the average of 2004–2013. To understand the impact of the assumption, the same calculation was also done while assuming incidence data prior to 2004 was the same as in the year 2004 and the year 2012, as the highest count of prevalence was identified in year 2004 and the lowest in 2012. To reflect the fact that the US life expectancies have increased over time and that women with oophorectomy had lower life expectancies than the general population [27], the probability of survival estimates were lowered from values in the US life tables by 0.5% when calculating the complete prevalence rates for prior SO.

To validate the prevalence estimates from the first method, we also used the BRFSS data to estimate the prevalence rates. In previous published studies, prevalence rates of prior SO were estimated by multiplying the prevalence rates of hysterectomy from the BRFSS data by the proportion of hysterectomy incidences with bilateral oophorectomy [2]. Similarly, we calculated the ratio of SO vs.

hysterectomy by age group from the KHCD data for years 2004–2013 and the weighted prevalence rates of prior hysterectomy by age group for those aged 20+ from the BRFSS data for 2008, 2010 and 2012. The prior SO prevalence estimates by age groups were the product of the ratio of SO vs. hysterectomy and the prevalence of prior hysterectomy from the BFRSS data.

2.5. Age-Adjusted Incidence Rates for Ovary Cancer

All age-adjusted rates were calculated based on the standard 2000 US population. To examine how the different formats of age groups in the background population impact age-adjusted rates, the traditional age-adjusted rates based on the 19 age groups in the standard Kentucky population were calculated along with the traditional age-adjusted rates based on the 18 age groups defined in the KHCD data. To calculate the corrected age-adjusted rates for ovary cancer, the standard Kentucky population data were corrected by deducting the number of women with SO derived through the prevalence estimates from the two approaches previously discussed.

All analyses were done using SAS Statistical software version 9.4. SAS (SAS Institute, Cary, NC, USA) was also used to develop programs to calculate the complete prevalence rates from the KHCD data. Statistical tests were two sided with a p-value ≤ 0.05 used to identify statistical significance.

3. Results

There was a total of 81,359 SO cases identified from the KHDC data during 2004–2013 (Table 1). The highest frequencies were found in the age groups 41–45 and 46–50. Very few cases were found in women with ages younger than 20 or ages older than 80. The number of SO cases from the inpatient files had dropped steadily over the study period and the number of cases from the outpatient files had increased. The overall SO cases had consistently dropped since 2003 (Figure 1).

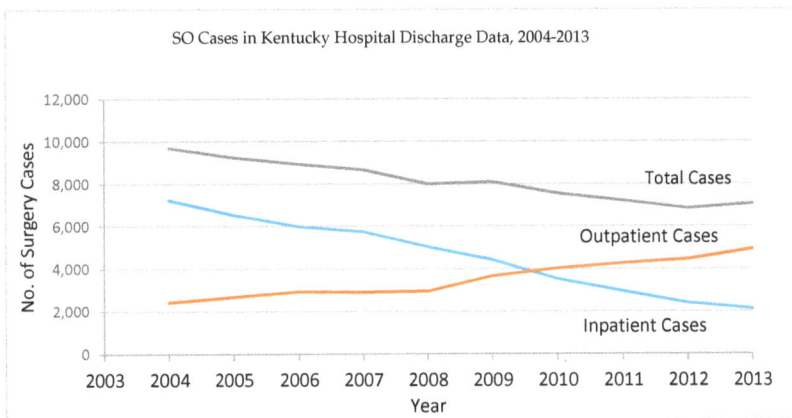

Figure 1. Trend of salpingo-oophorectomy (SO) cases from the Kentucky Hospital Discharge Data, 2004–2013.

Using the Counting Method, estimates of annual prevalence counts and rates by age group for the years 2009 to 2013 were calculated from the KHCD. Only results from the years 2009 and 2013 based on the assumption that SO incidences prior 2004 are same as the average in 2004–2013 are shown in Table 2. The results based on the assumptions that SO incidences prior 2004 are same as in 2004 or 2012 can be found in Tables S1 and S2. The prevalence rates increased by age and peaked at the oldest age groups of 76–80 and 81+. Because of the decreasing trend of SO cases, the prevalence rates had dropped from year 2009 to 2013. For example, the rates dropped from 27.4% to 24.4% in the age group 61–65 and from 42.1% to 38.1% in the age group 71–75 (Table 2).

Table 1. Salpingo-oophorectomy (SO) cases in Kentucky Hospital Discharge Data by age group, 2004–2013.

Year	Age Group																		Total
	0	1-5	6-10	11-15	16-20	21-25	26-30	31-35	36-40	41-45	46-50	51-55	56-60	61-65	66-70	71-75	76-80	81 and over	
2004	1	1	0	6	24	179	561	966	1482	2077	1919	987	445	356	265	202	142	79	9692
2005	0	1	1	7	24	191	542	887	1342	1999	1874	935	501	323	242	179	121	80	9249
2006	0	0	0	6	24	184	536	954	1308	1798	1662	894	500	365	277	201	142	87	8938
2007	1	0	1	5	31	193	500	833	1299	1669	1625	923	574	371	233	200	119	96	8673
2008	0	0	1	6	26	172	462	769	1119	1549	1512	832	486	382	306	179	124	86	8011
2009	0	2	0	8	38	147	500	771	1123	1530	1509	851	500	436	291	182	119	89	8097
2010	0	0	0	10	32	162	454	783	1075	1327	1373	828	479	384	265	198	112	75	7557
2011	2	1	2	12	40	155	411	764	1008	1241	1288	777	473	416	310	182	72	67	7221
2012	0	0	0	6	31	130	363	699	941	1185	1205	781	488	391	274	191	94	72	6851
2013	0	0	0	9	27	122	366	726	1031	1256	1188	748	518	425	307	186	103	63	7075
Total	5	5	5	75	297	1635	4695	8152	11,728	15,631	15,155	8556	4964	3849	2770	1900	1148	794	81,364

Table 2. Estimated SO Prevalence in Kentucky for year 2009 and 2013, by age groups *.

Age Group	Prob. of Survival	2009			2013		
		Population	Prevalence Count	Prevalence Rate	Population	Prevalence Count	Prevalence Rate
0	0.989	27,302	1.0	0.000	26,905	0.0	0.000
1-5	0.995	138,333	2.2	0.000	135,862	1.0	0.000
6-10	0.995	137,647	4.8	0.000	138,692	3.8	0.000
11-15	0.995	137,317	23.2	0.000	139,204	32.4	0.000
16-20	0.995	146,960	128.7	0.001	138,987	134.5	0.001
21-25	0.995	139,412	689.7	0.005	154,076	596.8	0.004
26-30	0.994	143,447	2624.1	0.018	137,250	2201.0	0.016
31-35	0.994	135,456	6206.3	0.046	142,561	5680.1	0.040
36-40	0.994	145,489	11,649.2	0.080	135,750	10,662.2	0.079
41-45	0.993	150,939	19,138.6	0.127	146,947	17,331.1	0.118
46-50	0.992	164,356	27,186.7	0.165	154,584	25,180.5	0.163
51-55	0.991	159,697	31,613.2	0.198	163,369	31,226.4	0.191
56-60	0.989	142,234	32,472.1	0.228	153,709	33,146.2	0.216
61-65	0.987	118,111	32,339.0	0.274	134,958	32,887.2	0.244
66-70	0.982	92,015	31,612.5	0.344	106,051	31,852.8	0.300
71-75	0.974	71,219	30,014.6	0.421	78,893	30,093.7	0.381
76-80	0.960	58,333	27,272.4	0.468	58,703	27,192.7	0.463
81+	0.911	84,869	39,805.1	0.469	87,494	39,812.0	0.455

* Assume SO incidence prior 2004 same as the average of incidence between years 2004–2013.

In Table 3, hysterectomy prevalence rates by age group were calculated from the BRFSS data for 2008, 2010, and 2012. The highest rates appeared in the age group 76–80. Ratios of SO vs. hysterectomy from the KHCD data varied from 65% to 103% by age group. The prior SO prevalence rates modified from the hysterectomy rates from the BRFSS data peaked in the age group 66–70 (50.7%) and were considerably smaller in the age group 81+ (42.5%) compared to the prevalence rates from the Counting Method.

Table 3. Estimated hysterectomy and oophorectomy prevalence based on the Kentucky BRFSS data and discharge data.

Age Group	Hysterectomy Prevalence Rate by BRFSS ^	Ratio of SO vs. Hysterectomy *	SO Prevalence Rate by BRFSS
21–25	0.000	0.902	0.000
26–30	0.024	0.723	0.018
31–35	0.076	0.665	0.051
36–40	0.120	0.649	0.078
41–45	0.196	0.719	0.141
46–50	0.256	0.879	0.225
51–55	0.379	1.010	0.383
56–60	0.415	1.033	0.429
61–65	0.461	1.021	0.471
66–70	0.513	0.988	0.507
71–75	0.517	0.963	0.498
76–80	0.532	0.900	0.479
81+	0.512	0.829	0.425

^ Estimated hysterectomy prevalence based on the KY BRFSS data, 2008–2012; * Ratio of SO vs. hysterectomy in Kentucky discharge data from year 2004 to 2013.

A total of 1403 invasive ovary cancer cases for years 2009–2013 were extracted from the KCR database. The age-adjusted rates from the standard Kentucky population show the rates 10.7 per 100,000 (95% Confidence Interval (CI) 10.2–11.3) for all ages (Table 4). To match the age groups defined in the KHCD data, the age adjusted rates based on the standard Kentucky population with modified age groups were also calculated. The corrected age-adjusted rates from adjusting the population under risk based on the prevalence estimates of prior SO from the KHCD data were 15.5 (95% CI 14.7–16.3) per 100,000 assuming SO incidences prior 2004 were the same as the average of the incidence in the years 2004–2013, 16.9 (95% CI 16.0–17.8) per 100,000 assuming the SO incidences prior to 2004 were the same as in 2004 (highest incidence), and 14.3 (95% CI 13.6–15.1) per 100,000 assuming the SO incidences prior to 2004 were the same as in 2012 (lowest incidence). The corrected age-adjusted rate from the BRFSS prevalence estimates of SO was 17.7 (95% CI 16.8–18.7), which is higher than the highest estimates from the KHCD data (16.9 per 100,000). Overall, risk population adjusted SO age-adjusted rates ranged from 33% to 65% higher than the rates from the standard population. We also included the age-specific rates for ovary cancer by various approaches in Table S3.

Table 4. Age adjusted rates for invasive ovary cancer in Kentucky, 2009–2013.

Type of Population Under Risk	All Ages				
	Population under Risk	N	Adj Rate	95% CI	
Standard Population ^	11,083,781	1403	10.73	10.16	11.32
Standard Population with Modified Age Group *	11,083,781	1403	10.73	10.17	11.32
Modified Population based on KCHD-Assumption 1 ~	9,630,865	1403	15.47	14.65	16.32
Modified Population based on KCHD-Assumption 2 ~	9,414,282	1403	16.88	15.98	17.82
Modified Population based on KCHD-Assumption 3 ~	9,847,449	1403	14.34	13.58	15.12
Modified Population based on BRFS †	9,009,436	1387	17.72	16.78	18.69

^ The standard 19 population age groups, 0, 1–4, 5–9, ... , 80–84, 85+; * Use the 18 age groups in the hospital discharge data, 0, 1–5, 6–10, ... , 76–80, 81+; ~Adjusted the standard population based on the prevalence rates from the Kentucky Health Claims Data; Assumption 1: Assume incidence prior to2004 same as the average in year 2004–2013; Assumption 2: Assume incidence prior to 2004 same as the average in year 2004; Assumption 3: Assume incidence prior to 2004 same as the average in year 2012; † Adjusted the standard population based on the prevalence rates from BRFSS data.

4. Discussion

In the efforts reported here, the rates of ovarian cancer were 33% to 65% higher when prior SO was taken into consideration than estimates from the standard population. Due to the limitation of data availability, the risk-population adjusted prior SO rates have rarely been calculated previously. In the current study, we used the KHCD data and the Counting Method, a modern statistical approach, to estimate the prior SO prevalence rates based on various assumptions and the risk-population adjusted SO rates. We also estimated the SO rates using estimated SO prevalence rates from the BRFSS data. The prevalence rates of prior SO from the Counting Method and the BRFSS data are different because of various assumptions and different data sources, hence leading to the variation of the risk-population adjusted SO rates. The results demonstrate the challenge to correctly estimate the rates because of the data limitations.

Compared to previous published studies with only one type of estimate [2], our study is able to provide a range of estimates that gives a more comprehensive view of the estimates. It is possible that the 0.5% survival deduction of probability of annul survival from the standard US life table was too harsh and caused the lower estimates of SO prevalence rates compared to the estimates from the BRFSS data. Using the ratio of SO vs. hysterectomy from the KHCD data to estimate SO prevalence rates from the BRFSS was likely biased as the ratio was based on incidence data, not prevalence data.

Ovarian cancer remains the deadliest gynecologic malignancy in the United States, being the 5th most common cause of cancer death in women. Over 14,000 deaths from ovarian cancer are expected for the US in 2016 [20]. Despite advances in operative care and chemotherapy, including the recent use of targeted agents for this disease, overall survival remains poor [20,28–30]. While ongoing research efforts continue to search for better treatments with which to combat this disease, another approach to improve survival is through screening and earlier detection of disease. The majority of ovarian cancer cases are diagnosed at advanced stage prior to the onset of symptoms. Pelvic exam has been shown to have limited value in detecting ovarian abnormalities, especially in postmenopausal and obese women [31]. Only 15% of cases are confined to the ovary at the time of diagnosis [32]. However, survival is much improved for women who are diagnosed at an early stage [26]. Therefore, efforts to increase the detection of early stage disease have a potential to greatly impact survival. Estimates that reveal the true risk of ovarian cancer will support efforts to screen for early stage disease.

Screening for malignancy has been highly effective for other common malignancies such as breast and cervix cancers [33,34]. Ovarian cancer meets criteria as a disease that could benefit from effective screening since it is the 5th leading cause of cancer mortality in women with proven improved survival when diagnosed at an earlier stage [20,26]. Screening has been studied in ovarian cancer, most commonly with serum Ca125 levels and transvaginal ultrasound (TVUS) or a combination of the two [35,36]. There have been four major trials that have evaluated ovarian cancer screening. The first of these is the prostate, lung, colorectal, and ovarian (PLCO) trial, which showed no benefit to screening [37]. There was a multicenter prospective randomized trial in Japan that compared screening with pelvic exam, serum Ca125, and ultrasound to routine care and saw an increase in the rate of optimal debulking in the screen detected cancers [38]. Optimal debulking has a known association with improved survival in ovarian cancer [39]. The University of Kentucky Ovarian Cancer Screening Trial (UKOCST) has been in progress since 1987 [40,41]. Over 45,000 women have been screened to date with TVUS. Detection of 47 ovarian cancers has been reported by the UKOCST and these women have improved five-year survival and are more likely to be early stage than women with clinically detected cancers [29,34,42]. Most recently, the results of the UKCTOCS randomized trial were published in the Lancet and have shown a survival benefit for screening [30].

Taken together, the available data from these four trials suggests screening works to detect disease at an earlier stage, which leads to improved survival. However, one of the most common criticisms of screening and the studies that have evaluated it is the lower positive predictive values, which are likely driven by the lower prevalence of this disease. Statistical calculations for predictive values vary greatly depending on the prevalence of the disease being studied, unlike sensitivity and specificity of a test, which remain constant. Thus, a test with inherently good sensitivity and specificity can be brought to improved predictive ability by narrowing the screening population to a high-risk group for which the prevalence is high.

One way to narrow threat risk population for ovarian cancer is by focusing on ages at which incidence is high. This has been commonly applied in previous screening trials and the results of the work reported here confirm the importance of age. In the present study, ovarian cancer incidence is highest for women over age 75, while the rate of hysterectomy peaks at age 65. Age continues to be one of the most important risk factors for ovarian cancer.

Given the importance of correct incidence to predictive calculations for screening programs and epidemiologic risk assessment, an accurate calculation of incidence is critical. An accurate assessment of risk is more easily determined in some diseases than others. If all subjects are at risk, then the calculation is a straight forward division of those diagnosed with disease by those at risk. This is not so clear in all diseases, however. For example, surgical interventions for unrelated problems can reduce the at-risk pool for certain disease sites. This has been demonstrated in the literature regarding endometrial cancer [5,43]. Correcting risk rates for endometrial cancer involves reducing threat risk pool (or denominator of the calculation) by removing those women who have undergone prior hysterectomy for a benign condition. Ignoring hysterectomy underestimates the risk for women who have not undergone that procedure and has also been shown to distort data regarding the distribution of disease [44]. Hysterectomy has recently been declining in nationwide statistics for the US, but remains one of the most common procedures performed in this country today, which alters the epidemiology significantly for uterine derived cancer risk [38]. Approximately 600,000 hysterectomies are performed each year in the United States, and around a third of all women have had the procedure by the time they turn 60 [45–47].

Salpingo-oophorectomy (SO) is even more difficult to quantify than hysterectomy. Many women elect to have their ovaries and tubes removed at the time of a hysterectomy that is performed for a variety of reasons related to primary uterine pathologies. Additionally, many women undergo bilateral SO either separate from a hysterectomy or at some time after a hysterectomy has been performed for a wide variety of primary ovarian or other conditions, many of which are benign. These include endometriosis, non-cancerous ovarian cysts or masses, risk reduction for genetic conditions, and for hormone reduction in breast cancer patients. The overall trend for SO in the US has been on the decline [48]. This decline coincides with the similar decline in hysterectomy rate. This decline may also be a result of data showing that surgical menopause prior to age 50 in women who never used estrogen is associated with increased all causes mortality [49]. Despite this, the rates of SO remain significant [42].

Given the robust number of women who have undergone SO, risk of ovarian cancer is greatly reduced for these women and importantly alters the epidemiology of risk for malignancy at this site on a population level. There are some important caveats to this reduction. Serous peritoneal cancers behave nearly identically to ovarian cancer and the risk for these cancers is unlikely to be altered by SO [50]. It should be noted that peritoneal cancer is quite rare. The protective effect of SO is illustrated in high risk women who have undergone prophylactic SO for BRCA mutation, and have achieved a drastically reduced risk of serous malignancy [16–19]. In one study, the relative risk of ovarian, fallopian tube or peritoneal carcinoma in women with known BRCA mutations after risk reducing bilateral SO was 0.04 (95% CI 0.01–0.16) [18]. Recent literature supports two separate types of ovarian malignancy, with separate pathogenesis [6–17]. Type 1 tumors are generally considered low grade malignancies that arise from the epithelium of the ovaries. Type 2 cancers generally include high grade serous malignancies that are felt to arise from the distal, fimbriated end of the fallopian tube. The fallopian tube is generally removed with the ipsilateral ovary in most procedures that are performed—few indications, if any, would preserve the tube if the ovary is being removed. Thus, protection from Type 2 ovarian malignancy is gained from ovarian removal in most cases since the tube is removed concomitantly (i.e., a salpingo-oophorectomy is typically performed rather than an oophorectomy alone).

An additional consideration is that there is a rising trend in bilateral salpingectomy rather than bilateral salpingo-oophorectomy, which allows ovarian preservation while still potentially reducing cancer risks [42]. The degree to which this procedure is as protective as SO has yet to be determined. The current study takes into account women having SO but not salpingectomy alone. An argument can be made to include these patients for future studies, which has the potential to further correct the underestimation of the prevalence of ovarian cancer for women who retain all portions of their adnexa.

Overall, the SO rate nationally has been reported to be declining. However, it is still common for women to undergo this procedure and greater than 40% of women still undergo bilateral SO at the time of hysterectomy [42,51]. This significant rate needs to be taken into account for estimating accurate ovarian cancer incidence. Failing to recognize and account for the population of women no longer at risk underestimates the incidence for the rest of the population. This was the driving motivation for the current study and the results confirm that incidence rates need to take surgical procedures into account. Incidence is certainly higher by all methods used for calculation in this study once SO was taken into account. This was true both with overall incidence across ages, as well as age-adjusted groups.

There is inherent difficulty in establishing the overall risk associated with SO. Prior studies have shown an overall mortality disadvantage for women who undergo premenopausal oophorectomy—prior to age 50—and never used estrogen therapy [43]. This decrease in lifespan may be attributed to changes in cardiovascular health and other important roles provided through the hormonal functions of the ovary. How this risk quantitatively translates to changes in expected lifespan on an annual statistical level is unclear. This study estimated decreased survival of 0.5% annually for women who had undergone premenopausal SO. However, these are estimates and the true annual change in expected survival is unknown. Even taking this into account though, all calculations still show that incidence is underestimated if SO is not taken into account when evaluating ovarian cancer.

The strengths of this study include the use of population level data and novel statistical evaluation to correct risk assessments in an important way for women with regard to ovarian cancer. A couple of limitations are worth noting. Most notably, this study is limited by the dependence on CPT and ICD codes for diagnosis. Actual operative reports or pathology reports were not available for confirmation of procedure performed. This introduces the possibility of inappropriate coding leading to incorrect inclusion (or exclusion) of patients in the analysis. In addition, newer ICD codes are more specific in that bilateral procedures are noted and were isolated for inclusion. This is important as unilateral procedures would not be expected to confer the same protection against ovarian cancer as the remaining ovary and/or tube could lead to a malignancy. Not all CPT codes separate unilateral from bilateral procedures and thus there is some uncertainty on the extent of adnexal removal with patients coded this way. Also, some hysterectomy codes are nonspecific as to inclusion of adnexal removal or not. Most notably, abdominal hysterectomy CPT codes can include patient "with or without" adnexal removal. Thus, using these codes can contribute uncertainty to the study as the true proportion of patient with adnexal removal with hysterectomy is not indicated by the code. About 30% of the procedures included in this study came from these questionable codes and the estimates for SO prevalence are likely over estimated because of their inclusion. Future studies can address these uncertainties by verifying procedures performed by complete chart review. This technique is time consuming and would limit the number of patients able to be studied, but is important for refining the exact risk estimates. The advancement of electronic medical records and more specific ICD coding will make this kind of confirmation more feasible in the future.

Additionally, because the KHCD data prior to 2004 are not available, the SO rates prior to 2004 were based on assumptions. This will certainly generate biases for the estimates. Although this study requires a range of assumptions, it is reasonable to assume the true estimate is captured within the variation of the estimates. There are no survival data available in the KHCD data, hence the 2010 US life table estimates with a 0.5% deduction were used to estimate the alive SO cases for specific prevalence date and age groups. How much bias is introduced and in which direction this bias goes is unknown. With increasing availability and reliability of health claims data, this approach will likely provide more accurate estimates in the future. The BRFSS data are limited by sampling biases, recall biases, and missing data. Overall, although we cannot provide specific rates for the SO estimates, we can conclude that the corrected rates of ovarian cancer were substantially higher when SO was taken into consideration than estimates from the standard population.

Finally, this study should be expanded to a broader national population as there may be important differences between the population in Kentucky versus other parts of the nation.

In conclusion, this study presents an important concept for correcting the underestimation of ovarian cancer risk for women who retain their ovaries and tubes. This correction has critical implications for the calculation of screening program performance in terms of predictive value. It is also critically important to refine the epidemiological assessment of the distribution of this disease and the populations at risk so that the highest risk groups can be identified, which will improve screening programs ability to reduce mortality from ovarian cancer while reducing harm from unnecessary interventions.

Supplementary Materials: The following are available online at www.mdpi.com/2075-4418/07/2/019/s1.

Acknowledgments: The University of Kentucky Biostatistics and Bioinformatics Shared Resource Facility was utilized for this project which are supported by the Markey Cancer Center (P30CA177558).

Author Contributions: Lauren Baldwin contributed to data summary review, abstract composition and manuscript construction; Lauren Baldwin, Bin Huang, Tom C. Tucker and Robert N. Ore contributed to concept development and manuscript organization; Tom C. Tucker and Connie White contributed to data access and collection; Bin Huang and Quan Chen contributed to statistical programming and performed statistical analysis; All authors contributed to manuscript preparation. The authors are solely responsible for subject development, data collection & analysis, and composition.

Conflicts of Interest: The authors declare no conflict of interest.

References

1. Ries, L.A.G.; Kosary, C.L.; Hankey, B.F.; Miller, B.A.; Edwards, B.K. (Eds.) SEER Cancer Statistics Review 1973–1996. National Cancer Institute, 1999. Available online: https://seer.cancer.gov/archive/csr/1973_1996/overview.pdf (accessed on 21 March 2017).

2. Merrill, R.M.; Feuer, E.J. Risk-adjusted cancer incidence rates (United States). *Cancer Causes Control* **1996**, *7*, 544–552. [CrossRef] [PubMed]

3. Wilcox, L.S.; Koonin, L.M.; Pokras, R.; Strauss, L.T.; Xia, Z. Hysterectomy in the United States, 1988–1990. *Obstet. Gynecol.* **1994**, *83*, 549–555. [CrossRef] [PubMed]

4. Lepine, L.A.; Hillis, S.D.; Marchbanks, P.A.; Koonin, L.M.; Morrow, B.; Kieke, B.A.; Wilcox, L.S. Hysterectomy Surveillance—United States, 1980–1993. *MMWR CDC Surveill. Summ.* **1997**, *46*, 1–15. [PubMed]

5.   Siegel, R.L.; Devesa, S.S.; Cokkinides, V.; Ma, J.; Jemal, A. State-level Uterine Corpus Cancer Incidence Rates Corrected for Hysterectomy Prevalence, 2004 to 2008. *Cancer Epidemiol. Biomarkers Prev.* **2013**, *22*, 25–31. [CrossRef] [PubMed]

6.   Alvarado-Cabrero, I.; Navani, S.S.; Young, R.H.; Scully, R.E. Tumors of the fimbriated end of the fallopian tube: A clinicopathologic analysis of 20 cases, including nine carcinomas. *Int. J. Gynecol. Pathol.* **1997**, *16*, 189–196. [CrossRef] [PubMed]

7.   Colgan, T.J.; Murphy, J.; Cole, D.E.; Narod, S.; Rosen, B. Occult carcinoma in prophylactic oophorectomy specimens: Prevalence and association with BRCA germline mutation status. *Am. J. Surg. Pathol.* **2001**, *25*, 1283–1289. [CrossRef] [PubMed]

8.   Cass, I.; Holschneider, C.; Datta, N.; Barbuto, D.; Walts, A.E.; Karlan, B.Y. BRCA-mutation-associated fallopian tube carcinoma: A distinct clinical phenotype? *Obstet. Gynecol.* **2005**, *106*, 1327–1334. [CrossRef] [PubMed]

9.   Medeiros, F.; Muto, M.G.; Lee, Y.; Elvin, J.A.; Callahan, M.J.; Feltmate, C.; Garber, J.E.; Cramer, D.W.; Crum, C.P. The tubal fimbria is a preferred site for early adenocarcinoma in women with familial ovarian cancer syndrome. *Am. J. Surg. Pathol.* **2006**, *30*, 230–236. [CrossRef] [PubMed]

10.   Kindelberger, D.W.; Lee, Y.; Miron, A.; Hirsch, M.S.; Feltmate, C.; Medeiros, F.; Callahan, M.J.; Garner, E.O.; Gordon, R.W.; Birch, C.; et al. Intraepithelial carcinoma of the fimbria and pelvic serous carcinoma: Evidence for a causal relationship. *Am. J. Surg. Pathol.* **2007**, *31*, 161–169. [CrossRef] [PubMed]

11.   Crum, C.R.; Drapkin, R.; Miron, A.; Ince, T.A.; Muto, M.; Kindelberger, D.W.; Lee, Y. The distal fallopian tube: A new model for pelvic serous carcinogenesis. *Curr. Opin. Obstet. Gynecol.* **2007**, *19*, 3–9. [CrossRef] [PubMed]

12.   Landen, C.N.; Birrer, M.J.; Sood, A.K. Early events in the pathogenesis of epithelial ovarian cancer. *J. Clin. Oncol.* **2008**, *26*, 995–1005. [CrossRef] [PubMed]

13.   Lengyel, E. Ovarian cancer development and metastasis. *Am. J. Pathol.* **2010**, *177*, 1053–1064. [CrossRef] [PubMed]

14.   Kurman, R.J.; Shih, L.-M. The origin and pathogenesis of epithelial ovarian cancer: A proposed unifying theory. *Am. J. Surg. Pathol.* **2010**, *34*, 433–443. [CrossRef] [PubMed]

15.   Crum, C.P.; Mckeon, F.D.; Xian, X. The oviduct and ovarian cancer: Causality, clinical implications, and "targeted prevention". *Clin. Obstet. Gynecol.* **2012**, *55*, 24–35. [CrossRef] [PubMed]

16.   Domchek, S.M.; Friebel, T.M.; Garber, J.E.; Isaacs, C.; Matloff, E.; Eeles, R.; Evans, D.G.; Rubinstein, W.; Singer, C.F.; Rubin, S.; et al. Occult ovarian cancers identified at risk-reducing salpingo-oophorectomy in a prospective cohort of BRCA1/2 mutation carriers. *Breast Cancer Res. Treat.* **2010**, *124*, 195–203. [CrossRef] [PubMed]

17.   Sherman, M.E.; Piedmonte, M.; Mai, P.L.; Ioffe, O.B.; Ronnett, B.M.; van Le, L.; Ivanov, I.; Bell, M.C.; Blank, S.V.; DiSilvestro, P.; et al. Pathologic findings at risk-reducing salpingo-oophorectomy: Primary results from Gynecologic Oncology Group Trial GOG-0199. *J. Clin. Oncol.* **2014**, *32*, 3275–3283. [CrossRef] [PubMed]

18.   Rebbeck, T.R.; Lynch, H.T.; Neuhausen, S.L.; Narod, S.A.; Van't Veer, L.; Garber, J.E.; Evans, G.; Isaacs, C.; Daly, M.B.; Matloff, E.; et al. Prevention and Observation of Surgical End Points Study Group. *N. Engl. J. Med.* **2002**, *346*, 1616. [CrossRef] [PubMed]

19.   Kauff, N.D.; Satagopan, J.M.; Robson, M.E.; Scheuer, L.; Hensley, M.; Hudis, C.A.; Ellis, N.A.; Boyd, J.; Borgen, P.I.; Barakat, R.R.; et al. Risk-reducing salpingo-oophorectomy in women with a *BRCA1* or *BRCA2* mutation. *N. Engl. J. Med.* **2002**, *346*, 1609. [CrossRef] [PubMed]

20.   Cancer of the Ovary: SEER Stat Fact Sheets. Available online: http://seer.cancer.gov/statfacts/html/ovary. html (accessed on 27 December 2016).

21.   Siegel, R.L.; Miller, K.D.; Jemal, A. Cancer statistics, 2016. *CA Cancer J. Clin.* **2016**, *66*, 7–30. [CrossRef] [PubMed]

22.   Capocaccia, R.; de Angelis, R. Estimating the completeness of prevalence based on cancer registry data. *Stat. Med.* **1997**, *16*, 425–440. [CrossRef]

23.   Gail, M.H.; Kessler, L.; Midthune, D.; Scoppa, S. Two approaches for estimating disease prevalence from population-based registries of incidence and total mortality. *Biometrics* **1999**, *55*, 1137–1144. [CrossRef] [PubMed]

24. Marriotto, A.; Gigli, A.; Capocaccia, R.; Tavilla, A.; Clegg, L.X.; Depry, M.; Scoppa, S.; Ries, L.A.; Rowland, J.H.; Tesauro, G.; et al. Complete and Limited Duration Cancer Prevalence Estimates. SEER Cancer Statistics Review, 1973–1999, 2002. Available online: https://seer.cancer.gov/archive/csr/1973_1999/prevalence.pdf (accessed on 31 December 2016).
25. Verdecchia, A.; de Angelis, G.; Capocaccia, R. Estimation and projections of cancer prevalence from cancer registry data. *Stat. Med.* **2002**, *21*, 3511–3526. [CrossRef] [PubMed]
26. Arias, E. United States Life Tables, 2010. National Vital Statistics Reports, 2014; Volume 63. Available online: https://www.cdc.gov/nchs/data/nvsr/nvsr64/nvsr64_11.pdf (accessed on 31 December 2016).
27. Contemporary OB/GYN: Bilateral Oophorectomy: Solving the Risk/Benefit Equation—Choosing candidates, Monitoring Outcomes. Available online: http://contemporaryobgyn.modernmedicine.com/contemporary-obgyn/news/modernmedicine/modern-medicine-now/bilateral-oophorectomy-solving-riskbenefi?page=full (accessed on 31 December 2016).
28. Oza, A.M.; Cook, A.D.; Pfisterer, J.; Embleton, A.; Ledermann, J.A.; Pujade-Lauraine, E.; Kristensen, G.; Carey, M.S.; Beale, P.; Cervantes, A.; et al. Standard chemotherapy with or without bevacizumab for women with newly diagnosed ovarian cancer (ICON7): Overall survival results of a phase 3 randomised trial. *Lancet Oncol.* **2015**, *16*, 928–936. [CrossRef]
29. Burger, R.A.; Brady, M.F.; Bookman, M.A.; Fleming, G.F.; Monk, B.J.; Huang, H.; Mannel, R.S.; Homesley, H.D.; Fowler, J.; Greer, B.E.; et al. Incorporation of bevacizumab in the primary treatment of ovarian cancer. *N. Engl. J. Med.* **2011**, *365*, 2473–2483. [CrossRef] [PubMed]
30. Ledermann, J.; Harter, P.; Gourley, C.; Friedlander, M.; Vergote, I.; Rustin, G.; Scott, C.; Meier, W.; Shapira-Frommer, R.; Safra, T.; et al. Olaparib maintenance therapy in platinum-sensitive relapsed ovarian cancer. *N. Engl. J. Med.* **2012**, *366*, 1382–1392. [CrossRef] [PubMed]
31. Ueland, F.R.; Depriest, P.D.; Desimone, C.P.; Pavlik, E.J.; Lele, S.M.; Kryscio, R.J.; van Nagell, J.R., Jr. The accuracy of examination under anesthesia and transvaginal sonography in evaluating ovarian size. *Gynecol. Oncol.* **2005**, *99*, 400–403. [CrossRef] [PubMed]
32. Jelovac, D.; Armstrong, D.K. Recent progress in the diagnosis and treatment of ovarian cancer. *CA Cancer J. Clin.* **2011**, *61*, 183–202. [CrossRef] [PubMed]
33. Whitlock, E.P.; Vesco, K.K.; Eder, M.; Lin, J.S.; Senger, C.A.; Burda, B.U. Liquid-based cytology and human papillomavirus testing to screen for cervical cancer: A systematic review for the US Preventive Services Task Force. *Ann. Intern. Med.* **2011**, *155*. [CrossRef] [PubMed]
34. Myers, E.R.; Moorman, P.; Gierisch, J.M.; Havrilesky, L.J.; Grimm, L.J.; Ghate, S.; Davidson, B.; Mongtomery, R.C.; Crowley, M.J.; McCrory, D.C.; et al. Benefits and Harms of Breast Cancer Screening: A Systematic Review. *J. Am. Med. Assoc.* **2015**, *314*, 1615–1634. [CrossRef] [PubMed]
35. Nagell, J.R., Jr.; Miller, R.W.; DeSimone, C.P.; Ueland, F.R.; Podzielinski, I.; Goodrich, S.T.; Elder, J.W.; Huang, B.; Kryscio, R.J.; Pavlik, E.J. Long-term survival of women with epithelial ovarian cancer detected by ultrasonographic screening. *Obstet. Gynecol.* **2011**, *118*, 1212–1221. [CrossRef] [PubMed]
36. Jacobs, I.J.; Menon, U.; Ryan, A.; Gentry-Maharaj, A.; Burnell, M.; Kalsi, J.K.; Amso, N.N.; Apostolidou, S.; Benjamin, E.; Cruickshank, D.; et al. Ovarian cancer screening and mortality in the UK Collaborative Trial of Ovarian Cancer Screening (UKCTOCS): A randomised controlled trial. *Lancet* **2016**, *387*, 945–956. [CrossRef]
37. Buys, S.S.; Partridge, E.; Black, A.; Johnson, C.C.; Lamerato, L.; Isaacs, C.; Reding, D.J.; Greenlee, R.T.; Yokochi, L.A.; Kessel, B. Effect of screening on ovarian cancer mortality—The Prostate, Lung, Colorectal and Ovarian (PLCO) Cancer Screening Randomized Controlled Trial. *J. Am. Med. Assoc.* **2011**, *305*, 2295–2303. [CrossRef] [PubMed]
38. Kobayashi, H.; Yamada, Y.; Sado, T.; Sakata, M.; Yoshida, S.; Kawaguchi, R.; Kanayama, S.; Shigetomi, H.; Haruta, S.; Tsuji, Y.; et al. A randomized study of screening for ovarian cancer: A multicenter study in Japan. *Int. J. Gynecol. Cancer* **2008**, *18*, 414–420. [CrossRef] [PubMed]
39. Bristow, R.E.; Tomacruz, R.S.; Armstrong, D.K.; Trimble, E.L.; Montz, F.J. Survival effect of maximal cytoreductive surgery for advanced ovarian carcinoma during the platinum era: A meta-analysis. *J. Clin. Oncol.* **2002**, *20*, 1248–1259. [CrossRef] [PubMed]
40. Nagell, J.R., Jr.; Miller, R.W. Evaluation and Management of Ultrasonographically Detected Ovarian Tumors in Asymptomatic Women. *Obstet. Gynecol.* **2016**, *127*, 848–858. [CrossRef] [PubMed]

41. Ueland, F.R.; DePriest, P.D.; Pavlik, E.J.; Kryscio, R.J.; van Nagell, J.R., Jr. Preoperative differentiation of malignant from benign ovarian tumors: The efficacy of morphology indexing and Doppler flow sonography. *Gynecol. Oncol.* **2003**, *91*, 46–50. [CrossRef]
42. Pavlik, E.J.; Ueland, F.R.; Miller, R.W.; Ubellacker, J.M.; Desimone, C.P.; Elder, J.; Hoff, J.; Baldwin, L.; Kryscio, R.J.; Nagell, J.R., Jr. Frequency and disposition of ovarian abnormalities followed with serial transvaginal ultrasonography. *Obstet. Gynecol.* **2013**, *122*, 210–217. [CrossRef] [PubMed]
43. Sherman, M.E.; Carreon, J.D.; Lacey, J.V., Jr.; Devesa, S.S. Impact of hysterectomy on endometrial carcinoma rates in the United States. *J. Natl. Cancer Inst.* **2005**, *97*, 1700–1702. [CrossRef] [PubMed]
44. Temkin, S.M.; Minasian, L.; Noone, A.M. The End of the Hysterectomy Epidemic and Endometrial Cancer Incidence: What Are the Unintended Consequences of Declining Hysterectomy Rates? *Front. Oncol.* **2016**, *6*, 89. [CrossRef] [PubMed]
45. ACOG. ACOG Committee Opinion No. 444: Choosing the route of hysterectomy for benign disease. *Obstet. Gynecol.* **2009**. [CrossRef]
46. Whiteman, M.K.; Hillis, S.D.; Jamieson, D.J.; Morrow, B.; Podgornik, M.N.; Brett, K.M.; Marchbanks, P.A. Inpatient hysterectomy surveillance in the United States, 2000–2004. *Am. J. Obstet. Gynecol.* **2008**. [CrossRef] [PubMed]
47. Wright, J.D.; Herzog, T.J.; Tsui, J.; Ananth, C.V.; Lewin, S.N.; Lu, Y.-S.; Neugut, A.I.; Hershman, D.L. Nationwide trends in the performance of inpatient hysterectomy in the United States. *Obstet. Gynecol.* **2013**, *122*, 233–241. [CrossRef] [PubMed]
48. Mikhail, E.; Salemi, J.L.; Mogos, M.F.; Hart, S.; Salihu, H.M.; Imudia, A.N. National trends of adnexal surgeries at the time of hysterectomy for benign indication, United States, 1998–2011. *Am. J. Obstet. Gynecol.* **2015**. [CrossRef] [PubMed]
49. Parker, W.H.; Feskanich, D.; Broder, M.S.; Chang, E.; Shoupe, D.; Farquhar, C.M. Long-term mortality associated with oophorectomy versus ovarian conservation in the nurses' health study. *Obstet. Gynecol.* **2013**, *121*, 709–716. [CrossRef] [PubMed]
50. Bandera, C.A.; Muto, M.G.; Schorge, J.O.; Berkowitz, R.S.; Rubin, S.C.; Mok, S.C. BRCA1 gene mutations in women with papillary serous carcinoma of the peritoneum. *Obstet. Gynecol.* **1998**, *92*, 596–600. [CrossRef] [PubMed]
51. Howard, B.V.; Kuller, L.; Langer, R.; Manson, J.E.; Allen, C.; Assaf, A.; Cochrane, B.B.; Larson, J.C.; Lasser, N.; Rainford, M.; et al. Risk of cardiovascular disease by hysterectomy status, with and without oophorectomy: The Women's Health Initiative Observational Study. *Circulation* **2005**, *111*, 1462–1470. [CrossRef] [PubMed]

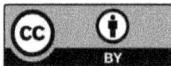

Review
Ten Important Considerations for Ovarian Cancer Screening

Edward J. Pavlik

Division of Gynecologic Oncology, Department of Obstetrics and Gynecology, The University of Kentucky Chandler Medical Center and the Markey Cancer Center, Lexington, KY 40536-0293, USA; epaul1@uky.edu; Tel.: +1-859-323-3830; Fax: +1-859-323-1018

Academic Editor: Andreas Kjaer
Received: 4 January 2017; Accepted: 7 April 2017; Published: 13 April 2017

Abstract: The unique intricacies of ovarian cancer screening and perspectives of different screening methods are presented as ten considerations that are examined. Included in these considerations are: *(1) Deciding on the number of individuals to be screened; (2) Anticipating screening group reductions due to death; (3) Deciding on the duration and frequency of screening; (4) Deciding on an appropriate follow-up period after screening; (5) Deciding on time to surgery when malignancy is suspected; (6) Deciding on how screen-detected ovarian cancers are treated and by whom; (7) Deciding on how to treat the data of enrolled participants; (8) Deciding on the most appropriate way to assign disease-specific death; (9) Deciding how to avoid biases caused by enrollments that attract participants with late-stage disease who are either symptomatic or disposed by factors that are genetic, environmental or social; and (10) Deciding whether the screening tool or a screening process is being tested.* These considerations are presented in depth along with illustrations of how they impact the outcomes of ovarian cancer screening. The considerations presented provide alternative explanations of effects that have an important bearing on interpreting ovarian screening outcomes.

Keywords: ovarian; cancer; screening; considerations

1. Introduction

Screening for different cancers, can appear similar; however, closer inspection reveals that there are considerable differences in approaches to cancer screening. This report focuses on the factors, issues and characteristics that uniquely distinguish ovarian cancer screening.

2. The Bare-Bones Basics of Screening

Cancer screening can be over-simplified so that it is conceived as the application of a test that discriminates malignancy. In general, the test for malignancy can be image-based or reagent-based. Image-based screening utilizes the identification of peculiar visual features not unlike correctly finding Waldo in an illustration that contains Waldo and other characters that may resemble Waldo to some degree [1]. Identification skills and sufficient time to complete the visual assignments are central to an image-based approach. Biomarker-based screening utilizes a chemical outcome which gives a result that discriminates malignancy, usually through a cut-off value above which malignancy becomes more likely. This approach can be thought of as asking the test for a "yes" vs. "no" answer about malignancy. This is best illustrated by the cut-off value of CA-125 (*cancer antigen 125*) for recurrent malignancy. However, one should be mindful that CA-125 becomes elevated by a variety of benign conditions [2]. Overlap in the outcome values of both malignant and non-malignant tests on both sides of the cut-off can occur with biomarker-based screening tests.

The key concept described above is "discrimination of malignancy". In simple terms this implies finding malignancy at a high rate, missing malignancy at a low rate, and testing non-malignancy as malignancy at a low rate. To do this, protocols that test screening discrimination must be designed to assess screening effectiveness.

3. Collecting Evidence to Examine Screening Effectiveness—Perspective Analysis for a Prospective Screening Trial

3.1. Consideration 1

Deciding on the Number of Individuals to Be Screened

After the screening tool has been selected, the first step is to make decisions about the size of the screening group framed against a time period needed to accumulate that number of screens. This time frame must be long enough to include a sufficient number of incident cases to give the incident portion of the study power because it is the screening detection of incident cases that can be expected to be at an early stage and demonstrate the clearest benefit from screening. In the Kentucky Ovarian Screening trial, approximately half the malignancies detected by screening were incident [3], and this suggests that the sample size predicted apriori by power analysis probably should be twice as large as a power prediction based on both prevalent and incident cases. For simplicity, incident cases can be defined as those detections that occur after receiving at least one normal screen. This sample enlarged for incidence should be able to distinguish screening effectiveness in prevalent vs. incident cases. A key issue is utilization of a standard of significance to determine power and test results in order to guarantee reproducibility. By comparing Bayesian hypothesis testing with classical hypothesis tests, it has been reported that thresholds for a significance finding should be changed to $p < 0.005$ [4], however, doing such would increase sample size, duration of the trial and ultimately costs [5]. Others favor less stringency and including assessments of actual costs, benefits and probabilities [6]. A potential solution is possible by balancing a weighted sum of type I (false positive) and type II (false negative) errors [7,8]. Bearing in mind that the present status of the UK Collaborative Trial of Ovarian Cancer Screening (UKCTOCS) [9] is an inability to detect a significant statistical difference in survival between screened and unscreened women, the chance of not detecting a difference between groups must be respected [10] by the doubling of sample size as outlined above. Although other factors have been enumerated that are responsible for research findings that are false [11], they do not mitigate the mistake of insufficient power based on choosing too low a level of significance.

3.2. Consideration 2

Anticipating Screening Group Reductions due to Death

Based on family reports and the Social Security Death Index (SSDI), 7.7% of 42,000+ participants in the Kentucky Ovarian Cancer Screening trial died after they began participating, with women over age 75 accounting for 70% of these deaths (Figure 1). Because of participants providing incorrect identifying information and due to the 3-year lag in listing on the SSDI, it is reasonable to expect an overall reduction in the screened population due to death of ~10%. Importantly, as the follow-up window extends to older age groups, a reduction in the screened population due to death of participants that can be followed for disease-specific survival will occur. This increase should be anticipated and used to adjust the group size predicted by power analysis.

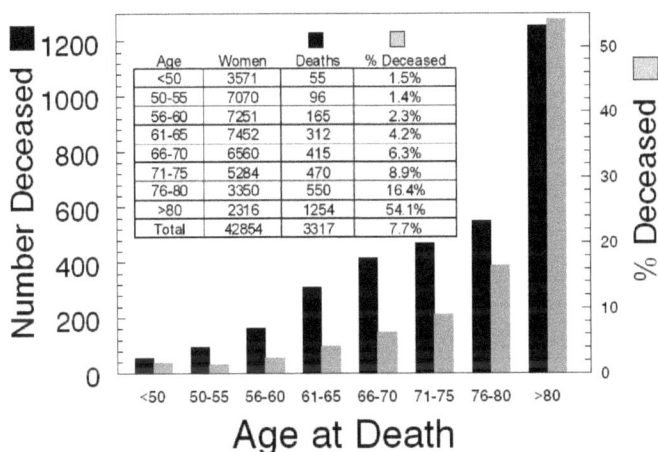

Figure 1. Age at death of screening participants.

3.3. Consideration 3

Deciding on the Duration and Frequency of Screening

The four major ovarian screening trials [3,9,12,13] used a periodic annual screening approach that accrued participants for 4.6–28.1 years and continued screening after enrollment for 7.7–28.1 years [14]. Two trials have employed a serial evaluation of abnormal screens [9,15]. Duration of the screening portion of the trial is a function of the sample needed and the resources made available to screen. A more difficult question regards frequency of screening. Screening high-risk women every six months has been practiced in the Kentucky trial without prior demonstration of benefit. The repeat screening interval after an abnormal screening exam is more subjective and has been performed at 3–6-month intervals on ovarian abnormalities that appear to be of low risk (cysts and cysts with septations) and at 4-week intervals for 3 months on ovarian tumors of uncertain malignant potential [16]. Annual follow-up for five years has been recommended for ovarian abnormalities that remain stable on several surveillance intervals of < 6 months [16].

A simplified picture of screening frequency is that women with a normal result be scheduled for annual screening, women with a result that is low risk for malignancy are screened more frequently and those with high risk for malignancy or with an abnormality of uncertain malignant potential are screened even more frequently. However, by what method can a result be assigned to one of these categories that minimizes subjectivity? Several characteristics are associated with an expected low risk grouping: (unilocular or septate morphology, morphology index (MI) = 4 or less, ΔMI less than 1.0/month, low-risk Assessment of Different NEoplasias in the adneXa or ADNEX score, absence of Doppler flow, CA125 (Cancer Antigen 125 <200 units/mL premenopausal or < 35 postmenopausal), CA125 stable/month, OVA1 (<5.0 premenopausal or <4.4 postmenopausal, OVA1 is the first multivariate index assay with FDA clearance), low-risk Risk of MAlignancy (ROMA) test, [17], absence of pelvic fluid), while others are associated with considering a high risk grouping (complex or solid morphology, MI >4, ΔMI (1.0/month or greater), high-risk ADNEX score, central Doppler flow, CA125 ($\geq$200 units/mL premenopausal or $\geq$35 postmenopausal), CA125 (doubling within a month), OVA1 ($\geq$5 premenopausal or $\geq$4.4 postmenopausal), high risk ROMA [17], pelvic ascites >60 cm^3). These characteristics have been discussed with more definition in the context of low- and high-risk groups elsewhere [16]. When a new screening modality is decided upon, one or more of these characteristics should be employed for deciding the frequency of its application based upon a potential for risk of malignancy.

An abnormality of uncertain malignant potential may be considered as a tumor of indeterminate status. Following these abnormalities for either resolution or worsening status presents a logical rationale. The Kentucky Ovarian screening Program has activated a protocol to decide if continuing surveillance or a decision-favoring surgery will be made based on findings [18]. In this protocol, four risk groups are defined. Risk Group A (MI_0 0–2) is considered for surgery if the MI increases by 2 or more in the first 4 weeks of observation or 3 or more in the next 12 months. Risk Group B (MI_0 3–4) is considered for surgery if the MI increases by 1 or more in the first 4 weeks of observation or 2 or more in the next 12 months (observation at 3 & 12 months). Risk Group C (MI_0 5–6) is considered for surgery if the MI increases by 1 or more in the first 4 weeks of observation or 1 or more in the next 12 months (observation at 3, 6, 12 months). Risk Group D (MI_0 7–10) is considered for surgery if the MI increases by 1 or more or remains unchanged in the first 4 weeks of observation. Thus, this protocol utilizes variable periods of observation that are determined by the level of risk determined initially (MI_0).

3.4. Consideration 4

Deciding on an Appropriate Follow-Up Period after Screening

An overly simple view of follow-up after screening is that it should extend long enough after the last participant in the screening trial has been screened to adequately assess the effect of screening on survival. However, a lesson learned from the UKCTOCS trial is that incident cancers occur after the first screen so that the follow-up for survival can be expected to be extended by one or more years. In the UKCTOCS trial, 4.6 years of screening accrual was coupled to 6.1 years of periodic screening and a final 3.1 years of follow-up. Secondly, over the course of a trial that occupies a decade of time, new treatments can be expected to be introduced that extend survival. Taken together, a longer follow-up extended to 10 years might be more appropriate for the UKCTOCS screening model to adequately assess the effect of screening on survival.

3.5. Consideration 5

Deciding on Time to Surgery When Malignancy Is Suspected

A 40-day tumor doubling time for ovarian malignancy has been estimated using the doubling of CA-125 [19]. While tumor doubling time may vary in different tumors, a 40-day doubling estimate is a good mid-range value [20]. Using this doubling time (Figure 2), comparative increases in size indicate that if the interval between a screen-detected abnormality and surgery is prolonged, tumor size will advance considerably. The mean volume of early stage ovarian malignancies (Stage I & II) detected by the Kentucky Ovarian Cancer Screening Program is 115 cm^3 (±26.7 (SEM)). This represents enlargement to about 75% the size of an orange (Figure 2 black dashed line) and upon removal is associated with significantly extended survival. After 90 days, malignant tumors with an initial volume of up to twice the size of the ovary will approach or exceed the size of an orange and this indicates that the time to surgery should be limited to well under 90 days after a screening is decided to be indicative of malignancy. Efforts in the Kentucky Ovarian Cancer Screening Program limit the time to surgery to less than 30 days to minimize the opportunity for an early stage screening detection to develop into advanced disease diagnosed at surgery. In contrast, the Prostate, Lung, Colorectal and Ovarian Cancer (PLCO) Screening Trial [13] allowed the time to surgery to extend for up to 9 months, a duration that would allow very considerable increases in tumor burden and the opportunity for the development of disease diagnosed at an advanced stage.

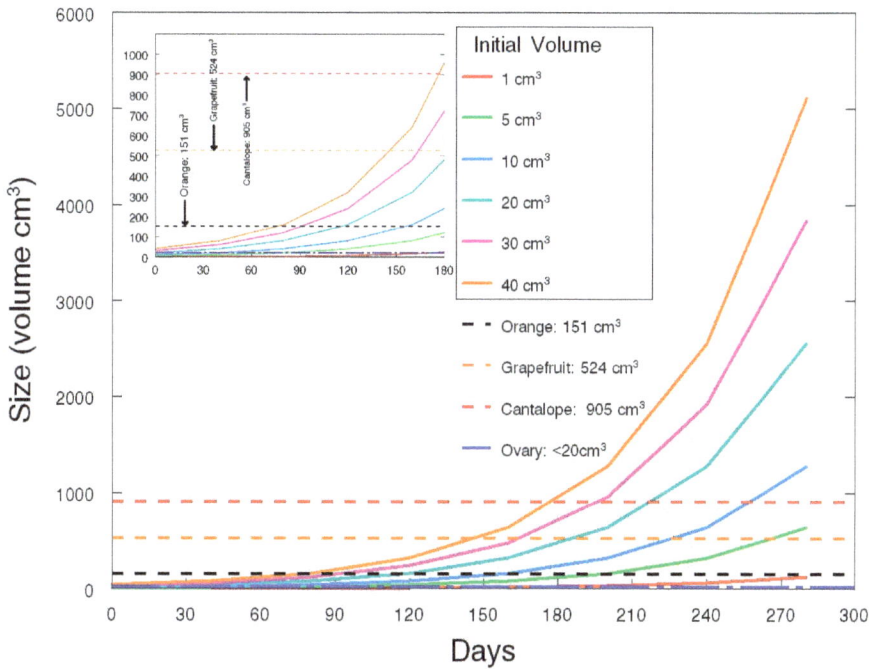

Figure 2. Ovarian Malignancy Doubling.

3.6. Consideration 6

Deciding on How Screen-Detected Ovarian Cancers Are Treated and by Whom

It has recently been recognized that better outcomes are achieved when ovarian cancer is treated by specialists at high volume hospitals [21–29]. No provision for treatment by specialists in high volume hospitals was included in the PLCO trial [13]. Consequently, it is likely that the treatment component of this trial under-performed the detection component and accounted for less than optimal survivals. In order to reduce confounding factors due to treatment that could be deleterious for survival, an ovarian screening trial should limit treatment to high-volume centers by a gynecologic oncologist adhering to National Comprehensive Cancer Network guidelines so that optimal therapy based on staging will be provided. Doing so may be particularly appropriate for early stage ovarian cancer in order that chemotherapy can be utilized in high grade tumors [29,30].

3.7. Consideration 7

Deciding on How to Treat the Data of Enrolled Participants

In the PLCO trial [13], the UKCTOCS trial [9,31] and the Shizuoka Cohort Study of Ovarian Cancer Screening (SCSOCS) trial [12], enrollment in the screening arm was subject to intention to treat (ITT) analysis so that participants were analyzed in the group to which they were originally randomized: "once randomized an individual was always analyzed", even if they were assigned to the screening arm, but never were screened or never received treatment. In this model anything that occurs after randomization is ignored, including non-compliance, protocol deviations, and withdrawal [32]. In contrast, in the Kentucky Ovarian Screening Program [3], only participants that completed the screening and treatment phases of the protocol were analyzed as a per protocol population. ITT analysis strongly favors preserving sample size so that originating power estimates continue to apply. The null hypothesis in a screening trial is that screening does not work. In the simplest sense, this null hypothesis is true if screening is falsely claimed to have a positive effect on disease, but positive screens cannot have a positive effect on disease if treatment is absent or sub-optimal. Individuals in the screening arm that do not receive screening and treatment will make the screening arm less distinguishable from the control arm, while individuals in the non-screening control arm that do receive screening and treatment will make the control arm less distinguishable from the screening arm. ITT analysis gives equal weight to each of these alternatives without testing for balance. Individuals who will seek out, schedule, attend and pay for screening are likely to occur less frequently than those who are assigned to the screening group but become non-compliant for receiving screens and treatment. This imbalance of never-screened individuals in the screening group is more likely to be greater than individuals who cross over to screening in the control group and will dilute the effectiveness of screening. This imbalance will not occur in a protocol-driven trial where unscreened/untreated individuals in the screening arm are censored, as well as individuals, screened independent of the protocol, in the unscreened control arm. In the PLCO trial, this imbalance consisted of 24 never-screened cases within the screening group, 21 untreated screen-positive cases in the screening group, and 8 cases in the screening group that were sub-optimally treated because they did not receive chemotherapy and accounted for 25% of the 212 malignancies reported in the screening group [13]. For the unscreened control arm, 25 untreated cases and 5 sub-optimally treated cases were reported or 17% of the 176 malignancies reported in the control arm [13]. No information was reported on how many cases in the control arm obtained treatment based on seeking access to the screening method. In summary, to test the question "Does screening work?" only cases of positive screens in the intervention group should be included that received treatment adhering to National Comprehensive Cancer Network guidelines, while the control group should identify and censor cross-over cases that obtained out-of-protocol screening.

The PLCO investigators decided to interpret the interval of protection conferred by screening to extend considerably beyond one year. Re-examination of the PLCO data by other investigators that limited the analysis to cancers detected within one year of screening showed that the survival in the screening group was significantly better than in the control group ($p = 0.0017$) and contained fewer Stage IV cases [33]. Thus, it is important to realize that malignancies that appear several years after screening should not be included in the intervention group, and should be censored as an "out-of-screening cycle" event.

3.8. Consideration 8

Deciding on the Most Appropriate Way to Assign Disease-Specific Death

Facile assignment of mortality due to disease is death that occurs with evidence of disease while under treatment for ovarian cancer, meeting the requirement used in both the PLCO and UKCTOS trials that *the disease process and/or associated treatments initiated or sustained a chain of events causally responsible for death.* Conversely, a sudden death with no evidence of disease is a death clearly due to other causes. Conditions for assigning disease-specific death are complicated when disease is evident and a sudden death occurs. Accidents, suicide, diabetic death, stroke and cardiac failure may be responsible for these complications. Difficult assignments of cause of death occur when reporting is incomplete. Both the PLCO trial and the UKCTOCS trial adjudicate disease-specific death differently [34,35]. The PLCO trial incorporated efforts to determine the underlying cause of death through periodic updates of questionnaires, cancer registries, and attempted contacts with next-of-kin and personal physicians (Table 1). Different procedures were used after the first two years of the PLCO trial to ascertain the underlying cause of death. The global resource available to the PLCO trial was the National Death Index which restricts the release of information until three years after any death has occurred. Admittedly, more information was available to the PLCO trial for screened cancers than for unscreened cancers and the control group [35]. The UKCTOCS trial had much greater global access to cancer and death registrations using the National Health Service (NHS) number of participants to access information from the Health & Social Care Information Center, the National Cancer Intelligence Network, Hospital Episodes Statistics, Central Services Agency, the Northern Ireland Cancer Registry, and the Hospital Episodes Statistical records (Table 2). To resolve the underlying cause of death, two pathologists and two gynecologic oncologists relied upon an algorithm involving disease progression (new lesions or increase in size of original lesions by imaging), clinical worsening, or rising biomarkers. Clearly the UKCTOCS had a more comprehensive access to death and factors related to cause of death through information arising in national health services.

Table 1. Mortality review in the Prostate, Lung, Colorectal and Ovarian Cancer Screening (PLCO) trial.

PLCO	PLCO	PLCO
Death due to ovarian cancer	The disease process and/or associated treatments initiated or sustained a chain of events causally responsible for death	Identify other underlying cause of death
Annual update questionnaire	Periodic	
Population-based cancer registries	Whenever possible	
Linkage to National Death Index	Periodic	
Obtained diagnostic medical records: Abstracted by registrars: stage, histology , grade, and treatment	Reviewers blinded to participation in screened vs. unscreened arm	Identify next of kin and personal physician
Underlying cause of death: first 2 years	Death certificate & relevant determinations underlying cause of death	Potential, ovarian cancer deaths, deaths of unknown or uncertain deaths were reviewed by at least 1 member of a panel of expertise (2 reviewers with discrepancies decided by a third)
Underlying cause of death: after year 2	Primary reviewer considered records without access to death certificate	If primary review disagreed with death certificate, a second expert reviewed record & death certificate. Disagreement triggered another independent review which led to a resolution by meeting or teleconference
Attempt to collect identical death information from both screen-detected and non-screen detected cancers	Screen-detected cancers will have more extensive information collected	Less information for both unscreened group participants & screened false positives

Table 2. Mortality review in the UK Collaborative Trial of Ovarian Cancer Screening (UKCTOCS) trial.

UKCTOCS	UKCTOCS	UKCTOCS
Direct communication with participants		
Postal follow-up questionnaires	3–5 years after randomization	
Diagnosis: England & Wales	Linked by NHS number to the Health & Social Care Information Center, the National Cancer Intelligence Network, Hospital Episodes Statistics	Cancer & death registrations
Diagnosis: Northern Ireland	Central Services Agency and the Northern Ireland Cancer Registry	Cancer & death registrations
Surgery outside the trial	Hospital Episodes Statistical records	
Underlying cause of death	Outcomes review committee (2 pathologists & 2 gynecological oncologists)	Final diagnosis based on algorithm: disease progression, (new lesions or increase in size of original lesions by imaging, clinical worsening, or rising biomarkers)

3.9. Consideration 9

Deciding How to Avoid Biases Caused by Enrollments that Attract Participants with Late-Stage Disease Who Are either Symptomatic or Disposed by Factors that Are Genetic, Environmental or Social

It may be possible to explain the failure to detect early stage disease in the PLCO trial in terms of promotions that attracted symptomatic women or women already with late-stage disease. If recruitment inadvertently allowed a biased enrollment of women who already were demonstrating clinical disease, it would certainly explain why early stage disease was not detected. Such a bias could also be contributed to by attracting nulliparous women or women with a family history of ovarian cancer. In contrast to the PLCO trial, the UKCTOCS ran a separate protocol specialized for women at elevated risk for ovarian cancer. Since screening is intended for detecting sub-clinical disease, post-hoc analysis should be performed that censors participants with clinical manifestations of disease when the screening tool is not needed.

3.10. Consideration 10

Deciding Whether the Screening Tool or a Screening Process Is Being Tested

Differences in the screening process between the PLCO and UKCTOCS trials have already been outlined here and in print [14,36] and are likely to have greater impact on outcomes than differences in the screening tools in these two trials. As an aside, completion of full human papillomavirus (HPV) vaccination is subject to age, rural vs. urban location, parental hesitancy/refusal and cultural factors [37,38]. In this example, which utilizes a very effective agent, effectiveness at the population level is limited by these barriers to utilization so that the role of the process assumes great importance even with a very effective vaccination tool. In summary, in a screening trial both the screening tool and the screening process contribute to the overall evaluation so that it is possible for a quite effective screening tool to be utilized in a flawed screening process with the result that overall outcomes are unimpressive. As part of this consideration, the control group is also process driven. If the control group is supposed to receive "usual care", such care could involve no visits to a care-giver as well as timed annual visits that are matched to the frequency of screening visits. In this latter case, the scheduled visits may provide a superior level of care that, based on information related by the subject, leads to imaging with CT or MRI and the potential to identify malignancy. Against this background it is not surprising that individuals in the control arm of clinical trials do better than the overall population.

4. Conclusions

Ten considerations are presented here that can impact the outcomes of ovarian cancer screening. Each should be considered for implementing screening processes and re-considered in post-hoc analyses as alternative explanations of effects that influence screening outcomes.

In addition, the consideration of ovarian cancer risk is appropriate and has been coupled to ovarian cancer screening. The United Kingdom Familial Ovarian Cancer Screening Study (UKFOCS) was begun in 2007 and included 4348 women that received annual screening for five years and follow-up for an additional 4.8 years [39]. The participants met the familial criteria for risk by having had a family member that had been diagnosed with ovarian cancer and would be considered to have a life-time risk $\geq$10%. A shift to early-stage ovarian cancer discovery was observed to result from this screening; however, it is too early to tell if an improved survival will be demonstrated in this screened group of high-risk women. Improved assessments of risk have now been defined based on mutations in $BRCA_1$ (Breast Cancer susceptibility gene 1: 39%–65% life-time risk), and $BRCA_2$ (Breast Cancer susceptibility gene 2: 11%–37% life-time risk) [40,41]. Additional germline mutations in $BRIP_1$, $BARD_1$, $PALB_2$, NBN, RAD51B, RAD51C, RAD51D [42,43] as well as MLH_1, MSH_2, MSH_6, PMS_2, EPCAM, (all associated with Lynch syndrome [44]), TP_{53} (associated with Li-Fraumeni syndrome [45]) and

STK_{11}/LKB_1 (associated with Peutz-Jeghers syndrome [46]) are related to moderately increased risk of ovarian cancer. With the number of germline mutations expanding, there has been support for population-based screening for all women before ovarian cancer develops [47]. Such a position would allow surveillance screening, surgical prophylaxis, or chemoprevention through oral contraceptives. However, utilization of these strategies must be weighed against potential problems (false negative screening, surgical complications, stroke, pre-mature menopause and increasing the risk of other cancers). Thus, with the list of associated gene mutations evolving, more women can be expected to carry some mutation pre-disposing them to ovarian cancer and overall will exceed the 15% of all ovarian cancers attributed to $BRCA_1$ and $BRCA_2$ [46]. In this context, some form of ovarian cancer screening/surveillance will have a role.

Conflicts of Interest: The author declares no conflict of interest.

References

1. Handford, M. *Where's Waldo?* Candlewick Press: Somerville, MA, USA, 2012.
2. Daoud, E.; Bodor, G. CA-125 concentrations in malignant and nonmalignant disease. *Clin. Chem.* **1991**, *37*, 1968–1974. [PubMed]
3. Nagell, J.R., Jr.; Miller, R.W.; Desimone, C.P.; Ueland, F.R.; Podzielinski, I.; Goodrich, S.T.; Elder, J.W.; Huang, B.; Kryscio, R.J.; Pavlik, E.J. Long-term survival of women with epithelial ovarian cancer detected by ultrasonographic screening. *Obstet. Gynecol.* **2011**, *118*, 1212–1221. [CrossRef] [PubMed]
4. Johnson, V.E. Revised standards for statistical evidence. *Proc. Natl. Acad. Sci. USA* **2013**, *110*, 19313–19317. [CrossRef] [PubMed]
5. Gaudart, J.; Huiart, L.; Milligan, P.J.; Thiebaut, R.; Giorgi, R. Reproducibility issues in science, is *p* value really the only answer? *Proc. Natl. Acad. Sci. USA* **2014**, *111*, E1934. [CrossRef] [PubMed]
6. Gelmana, A.; Rober, C.P. Revised evidence for statistical standards. *Proc. Natl. Acad. Sci. USA* **2014**, *111*, E1933. [CrossRef] [PubMed]
7. Jeffreys, H. *Theory of Probability*; Oxford University Press Inc.: New York, NY, USA, 1961.
8. Pericchi, L.; Pereira, C.A.; Pérez, M.E. Adaptive revised standards for statistical evidence. *Proc. Natl. Acad. Sci. USA* **2014**, *111*, E1935. [CrossRef] [PubMed]
9. Jacobs, I.J.; Menon, U.; Ryan, A.; Gentry-Maharaj, A.; Burnell, M.; Kalsi, J.K.; Amso, N.N.; Apostolidou, S.; Benjamin, E.; Cruickshank, D.; et al. Ovarian cancer screening and mortality in the UK Collaborative Trial of Ovarian Cancer Screening (UKCTOCS): A randomised controlled trial. *Lancet* **2016**, *387*, 945–956. [CrossRef]
10. Stokes, L. Sample size calculation for a hypothesis test. *JAMA* **2014**, *312*, 180–181. [CrossRef] [PubMed]
11. Ioannidis, J.P.A. Why Most Published Research Findings Are False. *PLoS Med.* **2005**, *2*, e124. [CrossRef] [PubMed]
12. Kobayashi, H.; Yamada, Y.; Sado, T.; Sakata, M.; Yoshida, S.; Kawaguchi, R.; Kanayama, S.; Shigetomi, H.; Haruta, S.; Tsuji, Y.; et al. A randomized study of screening for ovarian cancer: A multicenter study in Japan. *Int. J. Gynecol. Cancer* **2008**, *18*, 414–420. [CrossRef] [PubMed]
13. Buys, S.S.; Partridge, E.; Black, A.; Johnson, C.C.; Lamerato, L.; Isaacs, C.; Reding, D.J.; Greenlee, R.T.; Yokochi, L.A.; Kessel, B.; et al. Effect of screening on ovarian cancer mortality—The Prostate, Lung, Colorectal and Ovarian (PLCO) Cancer Screening Randomized Controlled Trial. *JAMA* **2011**, *305*, 2295–2303. [CrossRef] [PubMed]
14. Pavlik, E.J. Ovarian cancer screening effectiveness: A realization from the UK Collaborative Trial of Ovarian Cancer Screening. *Women Health* **2016**, *12*, 5–475. [CrossRef] [PubMed]
15. Pavlik, E.J.; Ueland, F.R.; Miller, R.W.; Ubellacker, J.M.; Desimone, C.P.; Elder, J.; Hoff, J.; Baldwin, L.; Kryscio, R.J.; Nagell, J.R., Jr. Frequency and disposition of ovarian abnormalities followed with serial transvaginal ultrasonography. *Obstet. Gynecol.* **2013**, *122 Pt 1*, 210–217. [CrossRef] [PubMed]
16. Nagell, J.R., Jr.; Miller, R.W. Evaluation and Management of Ultrasonographically Detected Ovarian Tumors in Asymptomatic Women. *Obstet. Gynecol.* **2016**, *127*, 848–858. [CrossRef] [PubMed]
17. Moore, R.G.; Miller, M.C.; Disilvestro, P.; Landrum, L.M.; Gajewski, W.; Ball, J.J.; Skates, S.J. Evaluation of the diagnostic accuracy of the risk of ovarian malignancy algorithm in women with a pelvic mass. *Obstet. Gynecol.* **2011**, *118*, 280–288. [CrossRef] [PubMed]

18. Elder, J.W.; Pavlik, E.J.; Long, A.; Miller, R.W.; DeSimone, C.P.; Hoff, J.T.; Ueland, W.R.; Kryscio, R.J.; van Nagell, J.R., Jr.; Ueland, F.R. Serial ultrasonographic evaluation of ovarian abnormalities with a morphology index. *Gynecol. Oncol.* **2014**, *135*, 8–12. [CrossRef] [PubMed]
19. Han, L.Y.; Karavasilis, V.; Hagen, T.V.; Nicum, S.; Thomas, K.; Harrison, M.; Papadopoulos, P.; Blake, P.; Barton, D.P.; Gore, M.; et al. Doubling time of serum CA125 is an independent prognostic factor for survival in patients with ovarian cancer relapsing after first-line chemotherapy. *Eur. J. Cancer* **2010**, *46*, 1359–1364. [CrossRef] [PubMed]
20. Willemse, P.H.; Aalders, J.G.; de Bruyn, H.W.; Mulder, N.H.; Sleijfer, D.T.; de Vries, E.G. CA-125 in ovarian cancer: Relation between half-life, doubling time and survival. *Eur. J. Cancer* **1991**, *27*, 993–995. [CrossRef]
21. Engelen, M.J.; Kos, H.E.; Willemse, P.H.; Aalders, J.G.; de Vries, E.G.; Schaapveld, M.; Otter, R.; van der Zee, A.G. Surgery by consultant gynecologic oncologists improves survival in patients with ovarian carcinoma. *Cancer* **2006**, *106*, 589–598. [CrossRef] [PubMed]
22. Earle, C.C.; Schrag, D.; Neville, B.A.; Yabroff, K.R.; Topor, M.; Fahey, A.; Trimble, E.L.; Bodurka, D.C.; Bristow, R.E.; Carney, M.; et al. Effect of surgeon specialty on processes of care and outcomes for ovarian cancer patients. *J. Natl. Cancer Inst.* **2006**, *98*, 172–180. [CrossRef] [PubMed]
23. Bristow, R.E.; Zahurak, M.L.; Diaz-Montes, T.P.; Giuntoli, R.L.; Armstrong, D.K. Impact of surgeon and hospital ovarian cancer surgical case volume on in-hospital mortality and related short-term outcomes. *Gynecol. Oncol.* **2009**, *115*, 334–338. [CrossRef] [PubMed]
24. Bristow, R.E.; Palis, B.E.; Chi, D.S.; Cliby, W.A. The National Cancer Database report on advanced-stage epithelial ovarian cancer: Impact of hospital surgical case volume on overall survival and surgical treatment paradigm. *Gynecol. Oncol.* **2010**, *118*, 262–267. [CrossRef] [PubMed]
25. Bristow, R.E.; Chang, J.; Ziogas, A.; Anton-Culver, H. Adherence to treatment guidelines for ovarian cancer as a measure of quality care. *Obstet. Gynecol.* **2013**, *121*, 1226–1234. [CrossRef] [PubMed]
26. Bristow, R.E.; Chang, J.; Ziogas, A.; Randall, L.M.; Anton-Culver, H. High-volume ovarian cancer care: Survival impact and disparities in access for advanced-stage disease. *Gynecol. Oncol.* **2014**, *132*, 403–410. [CrossRef] [PubMed]
27. Cliby, W.A.; Powell, M.A.; Al-Hammadi, N.; Chen, L.; Philip, M.J.; Roland, P.Y.; Mutch, D.G.; Bristow, R.E. Ovarian cancer in the United States: Contemporary patterns of care associated with improved survival. *Gynecol. Oncol.* **2015**, *136*, 11–17. [CrossRef] [PubMed]
28. Bristow, R.E.; Chang, J.; Ziogas, A.; Campos, B.; Chavez, L.R.; Anton-Culver, H. Impact of National Cancer Institute Comprehensive Cancer Centers on ovarian cancer treatment and survival. *J. Am. Coll. Surg.* **2015**, *220*, 940–950. [CrossRef] [PubMed]
29. Lee, J.Y.; Kim, T.H.; Suh, D.H.; Kim, J.W.; Kim, H.S.; Chung, H.H.; Park, N.H.; Song, Y.S.; Kang, S.B. Impact of guideline adherence on patient outcomes in early-stage epithelial ovarian cancer. *Eur. J. Surg. Oncol.* **2015**, *41*, 585–591. [CrossRef] [PubMed]
30. Vernooij, F.; Heintz, A.P.; Witteveen, P.O.; van der Heiden-van der Loo, M.; Coebergh, J.W.; van der Graaf, Y. Specialized care and survival of ovarian cancer patients in The Netherlands: Nationwide cohort study. *J. Natl. Cancer Inst.* **2008**, *100*, 399–406. [CrossRef] [PubMed]
31. UK Collaborative Trial of Ovarian Cancer Screening. Available online: http://www.isrctn.com/ISRCTN22488978 (accessed on 11 April 2017).
32. Gupta, S.K. Intention-to-treat concept: A review. *Perspect. Clin. Res.* **2011**, *2*, 109–112. [CrossRef] [PubMed]
33. Koshiyama, M.; Matsumura, N.; Konishi, I. Clinical fficacy of Ovarian Cancer Screening. *J. Cancer* **2016**, *7*, 1311–1316. [CrossRef] [PubMed]
34. Supplimentary Appenidix to Reference 9: Collaborative Trial of Ovarian Cancer Screening (UKCTOCS): A Randomised Controlled Trial. Available online: http://www.thelancet.com/cms/attachment/2049825434/2058773146/mmc1.pdf (accessed on 11 April 2017).
35. Miller, A.B.; Yurgalevitch, S.; Weissfeld, J.L. Prostate, Lung, Colorectal and Ovarian Cancer Screening Trial Project Team. Death review process in the Prostate, Lung, Colorectal and Ovarian (PLCO) Cancer Screening Trial. *Control Clin. Trials* **2000**, *231* (Suppl. 6), 400S–406S. [CrossRef]
36. Pavlik, E.J.; Nagell, J.R., Jr. Early detection of ovarian tumors using ultrasound. *Women Health* **2013**, *9*, 39–55. [CrossRef] [PubMed]
37. Sadaf, A.; Richards, J.L.; Glanz, J.; Salmon, D.A.; Omer, S.B. A systematic review of interventions for reducing parental vaccine refusal and vaccine hesitancy. *Vaccine* **2013**, *31*, 4293–4304. [CrossRef] [PubMed]

38. Wilson, R.M.; Brown, D.R.; Carmody, D.P.; Fogarty, S. HPV Vaccination Completion and Compliance with Recommended Dosing Intervals Among Female and Male Adolescents in an Inner-City Community Health Center. *J. Community Health* **2015**, *40*, 395–403. [CrossRef] [PubMed]

39. Rosenthal, A.N.; Lindsay, F.S.M.; Philpott, S.; Manchanda, R.; Burnell, M.; Badman, P.; Hadwin, R.; Rizzuto, I.; Benjamin, E.; Singh, N.; et al. Evidence of Stage Shift in Women Diagnosed with Ovarian Cancer During Phase II of the United Kingdom Familial Ovarian Cancer Screening Study. *J. Clinl. Oncol.* **2017**. [CrossRef] [PubMed]

40. Antoniou, A.; Pharoah, P.D.; Narod, S.; Risch, H.A.; Eyfjord, J.E.; Hopper, J.L.; Loman, N.; Olsson, H.; Johannsson, O.; Borg, Å.; et al. Average risks of breast and ovarian cancer associated with *BRCA1* or *BRCA2* mutations detected in case series unselected for family history: A combined analysis of 22 studies. *Am. J. Hum. Genet.* **2003**, *72*, 1117–1130. [CrossRef] [PubMed]

41. Evans, D.G.; Shenton, A.; Woodward, E.; Lalloo, F.; Howell, A.; Maher, E.R. Penetrance estimates for BRCA1 and BRCA2 based on genetic testing in a clinical cancer genetics service setting: Risks of breast/ovarian cancer quoted should reflect the cancer burden in the family. *BMC Cancer* **2008**, *8*, 155. [CrossRef] [PubMed]

42. Ramus, S.J.; Song, H.; Dicks, E.; Tyrer, J.P.; Rosenthal, A.N.; Intermaggio, M.P.; Fraser, L.; Gentry-Maharaj, A.; Hayward, J.; Philpott, S.; et al. Germline mutations in the *BRIP1*, *BARD1*, *PALB2*, and *NBN* genes in women with ovarian cancer. *J. Natl. Cancer Inst.* **2015**, *107*, djv214. [CrossRef] [PubMed]

43. Song, H.; Dicks, E.; Ramus, S.J.; Tyrer, J.P.; Intermaggio, M.P.; Hayward, J.; Edlund, C.K.; Conti, D.; Harrington, P.; Fraser, L.; et al. Contribution of germline mutations in the *RAD51B*, *RAD51C*, and *RAD51D* genes to ovarian cancer in the population. *J. Clin. Oncol.* **2015**, *33*, 2901–2907. [CrossRef] [PubMed]

44. Lu, K.H.; Daniels, M. Endometrial and ovarian cancer in women with Lynch syndrome: Update in screening and prevention. *Fam. Cancer* **2013**, *12*, 273–277. [CrossRef] [PubMed]

45. Shulman, L.P. Hereditary breast and ovarian cancer (HBOC): Clinical features and counseling for *BRCA1* and *BRCA2*, Lynch syndrome, Cowden syndrome, and Li-Fraumeni syndrome. *Obstet. Gynecol. Clin. N. Am.* **2010**, *37*, 109–133. [CrossRef] [PubMed]

46. Committee on the State of the Science in Ovarian Cancer Research; Board on Health Care Services; Institute of Medicine; National Academies of Sciences, Engineering, and Medicine. *Ovarian Cancers: Evolving Paradigms in Research and Care*; National Academies Press (US): Washington, DC, USA, 2016.

47. King, M.C.; Levy-Lahad, E.; Lahad, A. Population-based screening for *BRCA1* and *BRCA2*: 2014 Lasker Award. *JAMA* **2014**, *312*, 1091–1092. [CrossRef] [PubMed]

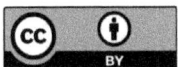

MDPI

Opinion

A Resident's Perspective of Ovarian Cancer

Christopher G. Smith

Department of Obstetrics & Gynecology, University of Kentucky Medical Center, 800 Rose Street, Lexington, KY 40536-0293, USA; christophergsmith@uky.edu

Academic Editor: Andreas Kjaer
Received: 5 January 2017; Accepted: 20 April 2017; Published: 27 April 2017

Abstract: Identifying, understanding, and curing disease is a lifelong endeavor for any medical practitioner. Equally as important is to be cognizant of the impact a disease has on the individual suffering from it, as well as on their family. Ovarian cancer is the leading cause of death from gynecologic malignancies. Symptoms are vague, and the disease is generally at an advanced stage at diagnosis. Efforts have been made to develop methods to identify ovarian cancer at earlier stages, thus improving overall mortality. Transvaginal ultrasound (TVUS), with and without laboratory tests, can be used to screen for ovarian cancer. For over thirty years, the University of Kentucky Markey Cancer Center Ovarian Cancer Screening Program has been studying the efficacy of TVUS for detecting early stage ovarian cancer. After 285,000+ TVUS examinations provided to over 45,000 women, the program has demonstrated that regular TVUS examinations can detect ovarian cancer at early stages, and that survival is increased in those women whose ovarian cancer was detected with screening and who undergo standard treatment. These results demonstrate the utility of TVUS as an efficacious method of ovarian cancer screening.

Keywords: ovarian cancer; screening; transvaginal ultrasound; quality of life

1. Introduction

As a first-year resident in Obstetrics and Gynecology, I am relating my perspective on ovarian cancer at this stage of my career. This disease has received modest attention during medical school and during residency. Having been to weekly didactics dedicated to this disease, as well as opportunities to scrub in on complex pelvic surgeries, I am beginning to understand more about the nuances of this disease process, its diagnosis, and management. Much of what I am relating here I have learned in my own efforts to eventually prepare me for a career in Gynecologic Oncology.

Cancer is the second most common cause of death among women in the United States of America and is the leading cause of death among women 40 to 79 years of age. Among the types of cancers affecting women, ovarian cancer is considered uncommon, yet it causes severe morbidity and mortality [1]. Abdominal ascites, bowel obstructions, venous thromboses, and adverse effects from chemotherapy are the realities faced by women diagnosed with ovarian cancer. Ovarian cancer is most often diagnosed at an advanced stage, which has led to investigations of screening tests to detect the disease at early stages. Transvaginal ultrasonography (TVUS) has been studied as a means to characterize and categorize adnexal masses. Since 1987, the University of Kentucky Markey Cancer Center Ovarian Cancer Screening Program has been studying the efficacy of TVUS for detecting early stage ovarian cancer. After over 285,000+ TVUS examinations provided to over 45,000 women, the program has demonstrated that regular TVUS examinations can detect ovarian cancer at early stages, and that survival increased in those women whose ovarian cancer was detected with screening and underwent standard treatment [2,3].

Histologically, ovarian cancer is any neoplasm arising from ovarian cells. Historically, these cells can either be those that line the surface of the ovary (epithelial) or those that originate from the ovary as non-epithelial cancers (embryonic or extra-embryonic (germ), hormone-producing, or structural cells [sex-cord stromal]) [4–8]. In recent years, numerous reports have proposed a unified hypothesis about the origin of high-grade serous ovarian cancer, implicating the Fallopian tubes fimbria as the point of origin [9–18]. In this hypothesis, invasive or serous tubal intraepithelial carcinoma (STIC) originating in the Fallopian fimbria is responsible for seeding the ovaries and peritoneal cavity with malignant cells [19]. However, STIC is not present in many high-grade serous carcinomas [20].

Ovarian cancer generally affects older women, the average age being 63 [21]. Ovarian cancer is the eleventh most common cause of cancer among women, with a lifetime risk of one in 70 to develop disease [22]. It is also the leading cause of death from gynecological malignancy. Nearly two thirds of ovarian carcinomas are diagnosed with disease located outside of the pelvis and thereby impose the consequences of advanced stage disease. Overall, the five-year survival rate for women diagnosed with ovarian cancer is 46%. When ovarian cancer spreads to distant sites, five-year survival decreases to 28%, and decreases to nearly 16% with Stage 4 disease [1].

2. Ovarian Cancer Risk Factors

2.1. Inherent Risk Factors

Over her lifetime, a woman has a nearly one in 70 chance of developing ovarian cancer [17]. However, certain risk factors confer an increased chance of developing ovarian cancer. Nulligravidity, or never becoming pregnant, can increase the risk for ovarian cancer. The basis for the increased risk is that repetitive ovulation can cause cellular damage, inflammation, and cellular repair, all processes that increase the likelihood of introducing DNA mutations. Multiple pregnancies, using contraception methods that interrupt ovulation, and ovulation suppression due to extended lactation can reduce the risk of developing ovarian cancer [23].

2.2. Genetic Risk Factors

The most significant risk factor for ovarian cancer is a strong family history of gynecological, breast, or colon cancers. These women generally have an underlying genetic predisposition to developing ovarian cancer and have mutations in tumor suppressor genes that prevent cancer [24]. Mutations that lead to the loss of function of tumor suppressor genes are recessive; therefore, they must be passed on by both parents to their daughter, resulting in an increased risk of cancer. However, in the case of ovarian cancer, there are mutations that are dominant, so that only one copy of the mutated gene needs to be inherited from either parent. BRCA-1 and -2 are tumor suppressor genes, specifically caretaker genes, that encode proteins involved in DNA repair that prevent the accumulation of mistakes encoded in DNA [25,26]. Ovarian cancer associated with BRCA-1/2 mutations is more indolent and affects younger women. Among women with mutations in BRCA-1, the risk of ovarian cancer can range from 39% to 44%, while the risk with BRCA-2 mutations 12% to 20% [27–29].

Lynch Syndrome is a disorder that predisposes women to right sided non-polyposis colon cancer and ovarian and endometrial cancers. There are five tumor suppressor genes mutations associated with Lynch Syndrome: MSH2, MLH1, MLH6, PMS1, and PMS2. Mutations in these genes are inherited in a dominant fashion, and result in increased microsatellite instability, or regions of DNA with incorrectly transcribed DNA. Ovarian cancer risk in women with Lynch Syndrome is six to 8% [30]. It is quite clear that women with inherited genetic mutations are at a greater risk of developing ovarian cancer, with a nearly three to fifteen-fold increase in risk for different gene mutations [31].

3. Clinical Presentation

3.1. Symptoms

Ovarian cancer is considered a "silent killer", meaning most women have no symptoms from the disease. Symptoms reported to be associated with ovarian cancer [32,33] are more often non-specific and associated with other conditions [26]. Sometimes, patients may present to their clinician with pelvic pain secondary to ovarian torsion. It is rare that any symptoms are associated with early stage ovarian cancer [34,35], and even when they do occur it is possible that they are coincidental. Women with advanced disease, however, are likely to have complaints of pelvic pain, abdominal fullness, early satiety, and bloating when tumor burden inflames abdominal structures.

3.2. Physical Examination Findings

A clinician may have an increased index of suspicion for ovarian cancer following their physical examination of the patient. A palpable pelvic mass, ascites with a fluid wave, or diminished breath sounds from pleural effusions can be identified on a physical examination. Rarely, a Sister-Mary Joseph nodule, resulting from ovarian cancer metastasized to the umbilicus, or the Sign of Leser-Trelat, which is an abrupt increase in seborrheic keratoses, can be indicative of occult cancer.

3.3. Ovarian Cancer Paraneoplastic Syndromes

Various paraneoplastic syndromes are infrequently associated with ovarian cancer. Hypercalcemia, usually due to increased levels of circulating parathyroid hormone releasing protein, can occur and cause altered mental status, increased thirst, urination, fatigue, constipation, and abdominal pain. Subacute cerebellar degeneration presenting as ataxia, dysarthria, vertigo, nystagmus, and double vision is due to cross-reactivity of antibodies to tumor antigens to cerebellar tissue. This condition usually precedes tumor occurrence by months to years, and can be associated with severe morbidity and mortality. Finally, Trousseau's syndrome, or unexplained thromboses, has been associated with ovarian cancer [36].

4. Diagnosis of Ovarian Cancer

4.1. Diagnostic Schema

If there is a high clinical index of suspicion, diagnostic evaluation can be undertaken. This begins with a transvaginal ultrasound (TVUS). TVUS is highly sensitive and provides morphological information about the ovary. Abnormal cystic findings on TVUS are broadly defined as simple or complex, with echogenic components in complex cysts more indicative of malignancy. Ultrasound findings can then be paired with blood tests that measure levels of tumor markers.

4.2. Tumor Markers

Discovered over 30 years ago, CA-125 is one of the most utilized biomarkers for ovarian cancer [37,38]. When circulating levels of the CA-125 glycoprotein are elevated, it is often indicative of ovarian cancer, although benign conditions like pregnancy, menstruation, endometriosis, and pelvic inflammation can also be responsible for elevated CA-125 levels [39]. CA-125 can be used to calculate the risk of malignancy index (RMI) for an individual patient. The RMI consists of a score assigned to TVUS findings, menopausal status, and CA-125 level. RMI values greater than 200 indicate high risk of malignancy [40].

A biomarker reported to be more sensitive for identifying ovarian cancer is HE-4, which is expressed on multiple organs but, surprisingly, not on the ovary. Elevations in HE-4 are found in nearly 100% of serous and endometrioid ovarian cancers and are sensitive in diagnosing early ovarian cancer. Compared to CA-125, HE-4 is not elevated in benign processes, allowing the biomarker to be specific for ovarian malignancy. The caveat for utilizing HE-4 is that normal values are not established. With the high specificity of HE-4, and the high sensitivity of CA-125, the utility of combining the two for diagnosing ovarian cancer has been implemented as the Risk of Malignancy algorithm (ROMA). The ROMA uses a mathematical formula utilizing HE-4 and CA-125 concentrations adjusted for pre- and post-menopausal status. Elevated ROMA values place women in a high risk of malignancy category. The ROMA serves as a good screening test that also has specificity for epithelial ovarian cancer. It not only detects more patients with ovarian cancer than the RMI, but also those with early stages of ovarian cancer [41].

In 2009, the Food and Drug Administration approved the clinical use of OVA-1, a serum test analyzing five biomarkers: CA-125, II-microglobulin (both elevated in ovarian cancer), apolipoprotein A1, prealbumin (transthyretin), and transferrin (which are decreased in ovarian cancer). Biomarker levels are used in a computer algorithm to provide a result between zero and ten and are stratified based on menopausal status. Patients with higher scores should be evaluated by a gynecologic oncologist because the complexity of their disease is expected to be greater than those with lower scores. To date, there are no studies directly comparing the performance of OVA-1 and ROMA [42].

5. Ovarian Cancer Staging

Once a woman is considered to be at high risk for ovarian malignancy, a referral to a gynecologic oncologist is made. Surgery is generally undertaken to properly assess the extent of the disease. An exploratory laparotomy through a midline incision allows for gross evaluation of the abdominal and pelvic cavities for disease. If staging of ovarian cancer is found to be necessary, saline is initially used to irrigate the pelvis and collected as "pelvic washings". This is followed by the surgical removal of the uterus, cervix, both Fallopian tubes, ovaries, lymph nodes that drain the ovaries (para-aortic lymph nodes), and the fat pad that insulates the intestines (omentum). Tissue is sent to the pathologist for final diagnosis of histological type, grade, and staging [31].

6. Treatment of Ovarian Cancer and Side Effects

6.1. Side Effects of Surgery

There are multiple side effects in the treatment of ovarian cancer. With surgery, potential risks generally include infection, hemorrhage, blood transfusion, pain, prolonged hospitalization, readmission, anesthesia complications, and death. Ovarian cancer surgical staging is often considered to be an "intermediate-complex surgery" and is associated with a 20% risk of morbidity and mortality occurring within the first 30 days following the operation [43]. Additionally, there is a ten to 15% risk of surgical site infections [44].

6.2. Chemotherapy and Associated Side Effects

Following surgery, most women receive some sort of chemotherapy treatment to eradicate any residual microscopic disease. More advanced stage ovarian cancer will have a greater likelihood of being associated with residual disease. Various platinum-based chemotherapy regimens have been used and are dependent on the stage of the cancer. These agents are not without side effects that can include nausea, renal and ototoxicity, myalgia, alopecia, bone marrow toxicity with resulting pancytopenia, mouth sores, swelling, redness, and chronic pain in the hands and feet (hand-foot syndrome) [45,46].

7. Psychosocial Effects of Ovarian Cancer

There can be considerable emotional and physical burdens associated with ovarian cancer. Anxiety and depression can develop from the distress over the pending removal of organs that represent a woman's femininity, motherhood, and sexuality [47]. Recurrence of disease is common, nearly 80% with advanced stage, serving as another nidus for stress. In a study from the Dana-Farber Cancer Institute, 56% of ovarian cancer survivors surveyed were concerned about recurrence [48]. Anxiety and depression is nearly two times more likely in women with ovarian cancer, and higher if there are other underlying health issues. Additionally, nearly 33% of ovarian cancer patients experience high levels of psychological distress [49]. The burden of ovarian cancer can be extended to caregivers. The Australian Ovarian Cancer Study Group investigated the effects of ovarian cancer on the quality of life of ovarian cancer caregivers. This study found that in the last year of life, caregivers had lower quality of life measures as well as higher distress than those who were not taking care of ovarian cancer partners. Additionally, mental and physical well-being worsened the closer their partner came to the end-of-life. The most reported unmet needs of caregivers in the last six months were found to be concerned with managing emotions surrounding prognosis, fear of worsening disease, balancing of both the needs of themselves and their partners, the impact of caring for their partner had on their career, and making decisions in an environment of uncertainty [50].

8. Ovarian Cancer Screening

8.1. Overview of Early Detection of Ovarian Cancer

Advanced ovarian cancer is associated with decreased survival, and increased morbidity with not only the disease itself, but also surgery and the effects of chemotherapy. A recent study found that if 75% of ovarian cases can be detected as Stage I or II disease, there would be a 50% reduction in ovarian cancer related deaths [3]. Therefore, there have been multiple investigations to improve detection of ovarian at earlier stages.

8.2. Disease Screening Principles

One method is to screen women for ovarian cancer. Disease that benefits from screening is one that is (1) highly prevalent in the population, (2) a major health problem, (3) has a significant preclinical stage during which detection by screening is possible, and (4) is significantly more curable at earlier stages. Ovarian cancer satisfies these conditions, but does challenge the condition of prevalence.

Screening for a disease is the process by which an asymptomatic population is evaluated for the likelihood of having the disease before there are symptoms or any indication of disease. Screening has two outcomes: positive (likely has the disease) or negative (does not have the disease). The ideal screening test will have:

A.   High sensitivity: the ability to identify everyone with disease who tests positive (true positive) from everyone with disease (true positives + false negatives). Ideally, a highly sensitive test will have a low rate of false negative results so the test rarely misses subjects with the disease;

B.   High specificity: the ability to correctly identify subjects *without* the disease (true negatives) from everyone without disease (true negatives + false positives). A highly specific screening test will have a low false positive rate;

C.   High positive predictive value: the portion of subjects with disease that tested positive (true positives) relative to all who tested positive (true positives + false positives), a value dependent on the prevalence of the disease;

D.   High negative predictive value: the portion without disease that tested negative (true negatives) relative to everyone testing negative (true negatives + false negatives), which is *inversely* dependent on disease prevalence;

E.   Low cost: to allow maximum test affordability.

Table 1 summarizes these terms and relates them to ovarian cancer screening.

Table 1. Statistical terms and definitions used in ovarian cancer screening [51].

Term	Screening Result	Findings
True Positive (TP)	Positive	Histologically-proven ovarian cancer
False Positive (FP)	Positive	Benign ovarian histology
True Negative (TN)	Negative	No evidence of ovarian cancer 12 months after a negative screen
False Negative (FN)	Negative	Ovarian cancer diagnosed within 12 months of a negative screen

Sensitivity = TP/(TP + FN); Specificity = TN/(TN + FP); Positive Predictive Value = TP/(TP + FP); Negative Predictive Value = TN/(TN + FN). Reproduced from [51] with permission from publisher.

Screening tests are compared to an acceptable "gold standard" test, which is usually a definitive diagnostic test. It is typically invasive, unpleasant, expensive, or impractical for wide use. Considered the best test under "reasonable conditions", the "gold standard" test provides 100% sensitivity and specificity [52]. Regarding ovarian cancer, there is no current "gold standard" screening test. However, TVUS performs with the highest sensitivity and specificity. A TVUS is performed with a 5–7.5 mHz vaginal probe that generates accurate images of the ovary used to detect changes in ovarian morphology and volume that are subtle and usually inappreciable on physical examination.

8.3. Ovarian Cancer Screening Trials

8.3.1. University of Kentucky Ovarian Cancer Screening Program

There have been four large ovarian cancer screening trials with TVUS as the primary screening modality, one of which is the University of Kentucky Markey Cancer Center Ovarian Cancer Screening Program. Originally initiated in 1987 by Dr. John R. van Nagall, this project has enrolled over 45,000 women, and investigators have performed over 280,000 scans. The project includes two groups: asymptomatic women ≥50 years old, and asymptomatic women ≥25–49 years old with a documented history of ovarian cancer in at least one primary or secondary family member. Both groups of women are compared to an unscreened control group of women from the same geographic area who received the same treatment protocols over the same period. The groups undergoing screening undergo evaluation based on an established algorithm (Figure 1).

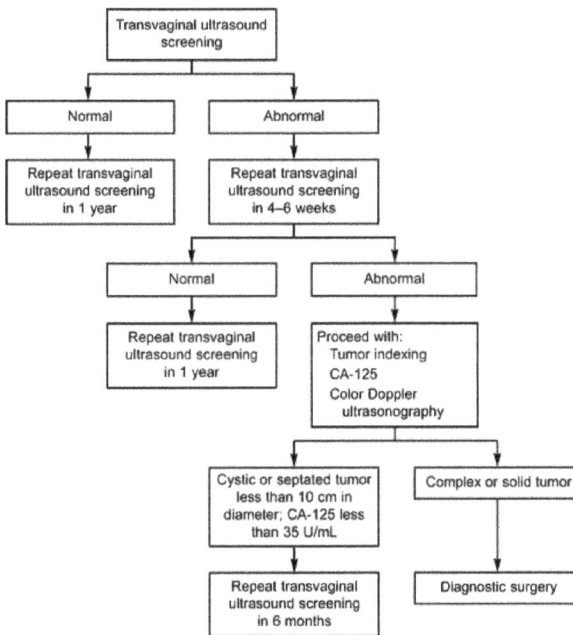

Figure 1. University of Kentucky Ovarian Cancer Screening Trial screening, evaluation, and treatment algorithm [53]. Reproduced with permission from publisher.

Using the algorithm, the detection of 53 primary epithelial ovarian malignancies has been reported [2]. Women who had ovarian cancer diagnosed by screening had earlier-stage disease (Stage 1 or 2) than those who did not receive screening (68% vs. 27%). The five-year survival rate of all women whose ovarian cancer was detected by screening compared to those not undergoing screening was

74.8% $\pm$ 6.6% and 53.7% $\pm$ 2.3%, a statistically significant difference. To date, the overall sensitivity, specificity positive and negative predictive values, and false positive rate are 86.4%, 98.8%, 14.53% to 20.17%, 99.97%, and 1.2%, respectively [54–57].

8.3.2. Prostate, Lung, Colon, and Ovarian Cancer Screening Trial

The Prostate, Lung, Colon, and Ovarian Cancer Screening Trial (PLCO) is a large, population-based randomized trial designed and sponsored by the National Cancer Institute starting in 1993 to determine the effects of screening on cancer-related mortality and secondary outcomes in men and women aged 55 to 74. Regarding ovarian cancer screening, women were assigned to undergo either annual screening with CA-125 and TVUS or usual care. There was no statistically significant reduction in ovarian cancer–related deaths between those screened and those who underwent usual care. There was a minimal increase in the detection of early stage ovarian cancer with screening than with usual care (22% vs. 21%). The five-year survival rate was 47.4% in the screening group compared to 36.0% in the group receiving usual care. The sensitivity, specificity, positive and negative predictive values, and false positive rate were 85.14%, 90.34%, 6.06%, 99.88%, and 9.6%, respectively [58,59].

8.3.3. United Kingdom Collaborative Trial of Ovarian Cancer Screening Trial

The United Kingdom Collaborative Trial of Ovarian Cancer Screening (UKCTOCS) trial recruited 200,000 women beginning in 2001 and randomized them into a usual care group, annual screening with TVUS group, or annual multimodal screening with CA-125 and risk for ovarian cancer algorithm (ROCA) group. The ROC utilizes an individual's CA-125 level profile (initial values and trends over time) and compares it to populations of women with and without cancer. The more a woman's ROC looks like profiles of women who have ovarian cancer, the greater her risk of having ovarian cancer [60]. Women found to have a high ROC scores were subsequently screened with TVUS per their algorithm. Results demonstrated an increased detection of low-volume disease (Stage 1, 2, and 3a) in the multimodal screening group than by TVUS alone (40% vs. 24%). There was no reduction in mortality regardless of the type of screening. Regarding the detection of any primary ovarian, tubal, or peritoneal cancers, the sensitivity, specificity, and positive predictive value for the TVUS group were found to be 84.9%, 98.2%, and 5.3%, respectively. The multimodal screening had a sensitivity of 89.4%, specificity of 99.8%, and a positive predictive value of 43.3%, respectively. When detecting primary invasive ovarian, tubal, and peritoneal malignancies, the sensitivity and positive predictive value of TVUS decreased to 75% and 2.8%. The multimodal screening was essentially unchanged, yet the positive predictive value decreased to 35% [61,62].

8.3.4. Multi-Center Japan University Trial

The final, large-scale ovarian cancer screening trial is the Multi-center Japan University trial. Over 80,000 asymptomatic women were divided into either a control group consisting of usual care following a physical examination or a screening group. Screening involved an annual pelvic examination, TVUS and/or transabdominal ultrasound, and measurement of CA-125 levels. The study showed that screening could detect Stage I and II disease at a higher rate compared to usual care (67% and 44%, respectively). Using the published data, the sensitivity, specificity, and positive and negative predictive values were 68.6%, 99.8%, 23.3% and 99.9%, respectively. The analysis of this screening protocol for the long-term effect on ovarian cancer mortality is presently in progress [63].

9. Life Is More Than Death: An Interview with the Husband of a Recently Deceased Woman Suffering from Advanced Stage Ovarian Cancer

In my short time in medical school and residency, I have made myself familiar with the pathophysiology of ovarian cancer, its treatments, the status of screening for the disease, and the survival curves that serve as the ultimate sterile summary of this disease. In all actuality, survival curves are the measure of time from diagnosis to death, conveying nothing more than the math of mortality. I have looked into the faces of women at various stages of this disease and have seen the suffering in their eyes as their mortality approaches them.

I felt compelled to convey only one story, a story that is much larger than the deaths due to ovarian cancer, because it is the journey on the terrifying road that women travel from their diagnosis to their death. I received permission to discuss the final stages of ovarian cancer with the husband and subsequent caregiver of a patient who died from ovarian cancer. To preserve patient confidentiality, identities are de-identified with pseudonyms.

9.1. Pre-Diagnosis Life

Mr. and Mrs. Johnson (pseudonyms) were college sweethearts who met through a mutual friend. Their first date consisted of a lovely bike ride across their college campus. Eventually, they wed and had three children. Mrs. Johnson primarily took care of their children and homeschooled them much of the time. Eventually, the children grew up and left home. She enjoyed working with her hands and loved embroidery, designing children's clothing, and creating smocking designs.

Mrs. Johnson took very good care of herself and never missed her annual gynecologic examinations. However, one day she noticed changes in her body. She mentioned this to her husband and said she "felt like she was filling up with water". Initially, they dismissed the complaint as something that would resolve itself. However, two days later, she again commented on how bloated she felt, and lifted her shirt, showing her husband how distended her abdomen was. She began to shake her hips, and they both could hear "water sloshing around her abdomen". Mrs. Johnson called a physician friend, who urged her to set up an appointment with her gynecologist.

At the discretion of her gynecologist, she underwent a CT scan and had a CA-125 level drawn. When her doctor entered the room with the results, he "had a complete change in his demeanor". Her CA-125 was over 15,000, and imaging showed some sort of gynecologic malignancy. Her gynecologist counseled her that she needed to be evaluated by a gynecologic oncologist and suggested she be evaluated at the Markey Cancer Center, located on the University of Kentucky Medical Center campus.

The gynecologic oncologist was certain she was suffering from at least Stage IIIC ovarian cancer and that a staging surgery was necessary. Surgery revealed extensive disease throughout the abdomen including involvement of the liver and diaphragm. A ureter obstruction required a ureter re-anastomosis by a urology consultation team. Post-operatively, she spent 11 days in the hospital, which was complicated by a right pleural effusion. The final pathology was consistent with high-grade Stage IVA papillary serous adenocarcinoma of the ovary arising from both ovaries. According to her husband, revelation of her diagnosis was "like being hit between the eyes".

9.2. Life after Diagnosis for Both Individuals

Though the chances of a five-year survival had been quoted as 15%, Mrs. Johnson had always been a strongminded individual, and she was determined to beat her disease. Chemotherapy options were discussed, and she elected to proceed with dose-dense carboplatin and taxol.

9.3. Life during Treatment for Both Individuals

Life during chemotherapy was a struggle, though she did not let those struggles dampen her faith and determination. Fatigue was the worst side effect from her chemotherapy to the point that she was unable to enjoy her usual embroidery activities. Faith played a large role in keeping her will to beat cancer alive. Her family and church members prayed constantly that she would not suffer from neuropathy in her hands so she could continue knitting, and thankfully, their prayers were answered. She had mild neuropathy in her feet with sparing of her hands.

Mrs. Johnson experienced recurrent pleural effusions, eventually showing evidence of malignancy and recurrence. She had the the lining of her right hemi-thorax removed, which did not show evidence of disease. Additionally, a new area of suspected malignancy on her spleen was evident on a repeat CT scan, along with a rise in her CA-125 to a maximum level of 4000. She received various chemotherapy regimens including, gemcitabine, Avastin with vinorelbine, taxotere, cyclophosphamide, and etoposide. External beam radiation therapy was utilized to address the malignant area of her spleen. She had 13 radiation treatments, but decided to decline any more radiation treatments because they caused more fatigue than her chemotherapy. Her cancer responded to the cyclophosphamide, but eventually her CA-125 began to rise. She declined further chemotherapy, and the topic of hospice was approached. She decided that she did not want hospice at that point.

9.4. Life during the Final Months for Both Individuals

The final months of Mrs. Johnson's life were filled with overwhelming difficulties resulting from her recurrent ovarian cancer. She suffered greatly from recurrent pleural effusions and abdominal ascites. She had nearly eight liters of ascites removed as an outpatient. She would continue to have paracenteses whenever she became symptomatic. She decided to resume chemotherapy treatment with etoposide. Two days later, she was admitted to the hospital with chemotherapy induced nausea and vomiting. She was discharged after five days, but was readmitted for intractable symptoms. She wanted to have a Denver drain placed to allow personal drainage of her ascites whenever she was symptomatic. This improved her quality of life considerably.

However, she suffered another setback when she was diagnosed with a small bowel obstruction. She elected to forego aggressive surgical treatment to address the obstruction and decided instead to go home to be treated with intravenous fluids. The topic of hospice was brought up multiple times, but she did not want to give in to her cancer. She was unable to tolerate any food, but she was determined to eat. The thought of food became an obsession, as she would "watch cooking shows and read every page of every cookbook in her kitchen". She developed a routine of self-induced emesis in the morning and evenings so that she could at least eat something. She continued to be symptomatic from her small bowel obstruction, utilizing outpatient intravenous fluid hydration and electrolyte replacements. Through all of this, she still declined hospice, with hope still alive of overcoming her disease.

Mrs. Johnson died in November 2016. From the time of diagnosis, she lived 33 months, underwent 66 chemotherapy treatments with 10 different chemotherapy agents, 13 external radiation treatments, five thoracenteses to relieve recurrent pleural effusions, and four paracentesis procedures that removed nearly eight liters of ascites. Mrs. Johnson did not live without pain, nor die without immense suffering.

9.5. Feelings of the Family (Husband) after the Woman's Death

Mrs. Johnson's family had a very peaceful Thanksgiving with her son and his wife assuming the cooking responsibilities that Mrs. Johnson had traditionally performed. Christmas was "a 'new' Christmas, but not a sad one". Mr. Johnson said that he did not regret anything about his wife's fight with cancer, and though it was the most terrible time for them, they would do nothing different if they had to go through it again.

10. Conclusions

It is estimated that a woman's lifetime risk of developing ovarian cancer is one in 70. Many ovarian cancers are diagnosed at an advanced stage, with only 15% of cases diagnosed in early stages. Ovarian cancer screening trials have attempted to diagnose women with early stage disease because survival is significantly greater in those patients. With screening programs like the University of Kentucky Markey Cancer Center Ovarian Cancer Screening Program, transvaginal ultrasound is effective for discovering early stage ovarian cancer. With continued efforts and determination, more ovarian cancers can be diagnosed at earlier, more curable stages, avoiding the pain and suffering associated with advanced stage disease like that endured by Mrs. Johnson.

Conflicts of Interest: The author declares no conflict of interest.

References

1. Siegel, R.L.; Miller, K.D.; Jemal, A. Cancer statistics, 2016. *Cancer J. Clin.* **2016**, *66*, 7–30. [CrossRef] [PubMed]
2. Van Nagell, J.R.; Miller, R.W.; DeSimone, C.P.; Ueland, F.R.; Podzielinski, I.; Goodrich, S.T.; Elder, J.W.; Huang, B.; Kryscio, R.J.; Pavlik, E.J. Long-term survival of women with epithelial ovarian cancer detected by ultrasonographic screening. *Obstet. Gynecol.* **2011**, *118*, 1212–1221. [CrossRef] [PubMed]
3. Van Nagell, J.R.; Pavlik, E.J. Ovarian cancer screening. *Clin. Obstet. Gynecol.* **2012**, *55*, 43–51. [CrossRef] [PubMed]
4. Bridgewater, J.A.; Rustin, G.J.S. Management of Non-Epithelial Ovarian Tumours. *Oncology* **1999**, *57*, 89–98. [CrossRef] [PubMed]
5. Sundar, S.; Neal, R.D.; Kehoe, S. Diagnosis of ovarian cancer. *BMJ* **2015**, *351*, h4443. [CrossRef] [PubMed]
6. Boussios, S.; Zarkavelis, G.; Seraj, E.; Zerdes, I.; Tatsi, K.; Pentheroudakis, G. Non-epithelial Ovarian Cancer: Elucidating Uncommon Gynaecological Malignancies. *Anticancer Res.* **2016**, *36*, 5031–5042. [CrossRef] [PubMed]
7. Karnezis, A.N.; Cho, K.R.; Gilks, B.; Pearce, C.L.; Huntsman, D.G. The disparate origins of ovarian cancers: Pathogenesis and prevention strategies. *Nat. Rev. Cancer* **2017**, *17*, 65–74. [CrossRef] [PubMed]
8. National Comprehensive Cancer Network. Ovarian Cancer Including Fallopian Tube Cancer and Primary Peritoneal Cancer (Version 1.2016). OV-D. Available online: https://www.nccn.org/professionals/physician_gls/pdf/ovarian.pdf (accessed on 4 November 2017).
9. Alvarado-Cabrero, I.; Navani, S.S.; Young, R.H.; Scully, R.E. Tumors of the Fimbriated End of the Fallopian Tube: A Clinicopathologic Analysis of 20 Cases, Including Nine Carcinomas. *Int. J. Gynecol. Pathol.* **1997**, *16*, 189–196. [CrossRef] [PubMed]
10. Colgan, T.J.; Murphy, J.; Cole, D.E.; Narod, S.; Rosen, B. Occult Carcinoma in Prophylactic Oophorectomy Specimens: Prevalence and Association with BRCA Germline Mutation Status. *Am. J. Surg. Pathol.* **2001**, *25*, 1283–1289. [CrossRef] [PubMed]
11. Cass, I.; Holschneider, C.; Datta, N.; Barbuto, D.; Walts, A.E.; Karlan, B.Y. BRCA-Mutation-Associated Fallopian Tube Carcinoma: A Distinct Clinical Phenotype? *Obstet. Gynecol.* **2005**, *106*, 1327–1334. [CrossRef] [PubMed]
12. Medeiros, F.; Muto, M.G.; Lee, Y.; Elvin, J.A.; Callahan, M.J.; Feltmate, C.; Garber, J.E.; Cramer, D.W.; Crum, C.P. The Tubal Fimbria Is a Preferred Site for Early Adenocarcinoma in Women With Familial Ovarian Cancer Syndrome. *Am. J. Surg. Pathol.* **2006**, *30*, 230–236. [CrossRef] [PubMed]
13. Kindelberger, D.W.; Lee, Y.; Miron, A.; Hirsch, M.S.; Feltmate, C.; Medeiros, F.; Callahan, M.J.; Garner, E.O.; Gordon, R.W.; Birch, C.; et al. Intraepithelial Carcinoma of the Fimbriae and Pelvic Serous Carcinoma: Evidence for a Causal Relationship. *Am. J. Surg. Pathol.* **2007**, *31*, 161–169. [CrossRef] [PubMed]
14. Crum, C.R.; Drapkin, R.; Miron, A.; Ince, T.A.; Muto, M.; Kindelberger, D.W.; Lee, Y. The distal fallopian tube: A new model for pelvic serous carcinogenesis. *Curr. Opin. Obstet. Gynecol.* **2007**, *19*, 3–9. [CrossRef] [PubMed]
15. Landen, C.N.; Birrer, M.J.; Sood, A.K. Early Events in the Pathogenesis of Epithelial Ovarian Cancer. *J. Clin. Oncol.* **2008**, *26*, 995–1005. [CrossRef] [PubMed]
16. Lengyel, E. Ovarian Cancer Development and Metastasis. *Am. J. Pathol.* **2010**, *177*, 1053–1064. [CrossRef] [PubMed]
17. Kurman, R.J.; Shih, L.M. The Origin and Pathogenesis of Epithelial Ovarian Cancer: A Proposed Unifying Theory. *Am. J. Surg. Pathol.* **2010**, *34*, 433–443. [CrossRef] [PubMed]
18. Crum, C.P.; Mckeon, F.D.; Xian, X. The Oviduct and Ovarian Cancer: Causality, Clinical Implications, and "Targeted Prevention". *Clin. Obstet. Gynecol.* **2012**, *55*, 24–35. [CrossRef] [PubMed]
19. Nezhat, F.R.; Aposto, R.l.; Nezha, C.T.; Pejovic, T. New insights in the pathophysiology of ovarian cancer and implications for screening and prevention. *Am. J. Obstet. Gynecol.* **2015**, *213*, 262–267. [CrossRef] [PubMed]
20. Schneider, S.; Heikaus, S.; Harter, P.; Heitz, F.; Grimm, C.; Ataseven, B.; Prader, S.; Kurzeder, C.; Ebel, T.; Traut, A.; et al. Serous Tubal Intraepithelial Carcinoma Associated With Extraovarian Metastases. *Int. J. Gynecol. Cancer* **2017**, *27*, 444–451. [CrossRef] [PubMed]
21. Surveillance, Epidemiology, and End Results (SEER) Program. Cancer of the Ovary—SEER Stat Facts Sheet. National Cancer Institute, DCCPS, Surveillance Research Program, Surveillance Systems Branch. Available online: https://seer.cancer.gov/statfacts/html/ovary.html (accessed on 9 November 2016).
22. Cancer of the Ovary: SEER Stat Fact Sheets. Available online: http://seer.cancer.gov/statfacts/html/ovary.html (accessed on 27 December 2016).
23. Webb, P.M.; Jordan, S.J. Epidemiology of epithelial ovarian cancer. *Best Pract. Res. Clin. Obstet. Gynaecol.* **2016**. [CrossRef] [PubMed]
24. Weinberg, R.A. *The Biology of Cancer*; Garland Science: New York, NJ, USA, 2014; Volume 231.

25. Duncan, J.A.; Reeves, J.R.; Cooke, T.G. BRCA1 and BRCA2 proteins: Roles in health and disease. *Mol. Pathol.* **1998**, *51*, 237–247. [CrossRef] [PubMed]
26. Yoshida, K.; Miki, Y. Role of BRCA1 and BRCA2 as regulators of DNA repair, transcription, and cell cycle in response to DNA damage. *Cancer Sci.* **2004**, *95*, 866–871. [CrossRef] [PubMed]
27. American College of Obstetricians and Gynecologists. *Hereditary Breast and Ovarian Cancer Syndrome*; ACOG Practice Bulletin No. 103; American College of Obstetricians and Gynecologists: Washington, DC, USA, 2009; Volume 113, pp. 957–966.
28. Antoniou, A.; Pharoah, P.D.P.; Narod, S.; Risch, H.A.; Eyfjord, J.E.; Hopper, J.L.; Loman, N.; Olsson, H.; Johannsson, O.; Borg, A.; et al. Average Risks of Breast and Ovarian Cancer Associated with BRCA1 or BRCA2 Mutations Detected in Case Series Unselected for Family History: A Combined Analysis of 22 Studies. *Am. J. Hum. Genet.* **2003**, *72*, 1117–1130. [CrossRef] [PubMed]
29. Brose, M.S.; Rebbeck, T.R.; Calzone, K.A.; Stopfer, J.E.; Nathanson, K.L.; Weber, B.L. Cancer Risk Estimates for BRCA1 Mutation Carriers Identified in a Risk Evaluation Program. *J. Natl. Cancer Inst.* **2002**, *94*, 1365–1372. [CrossRef] [PubMed]
30. American College of Obstetricians and Gynecologists. *Lynch Syndrome*; Practice Bulletin No. 147; American College of Obstetricians and Gynecologists: Washington, DC, USA, 2014; Volume 124, pp. 1042–1054.
31. National Academies of Sciences, Engineering, and Medicine. *Ovarian Cancers: Evolving Paradigms in Research and Care*; The National Academies Press: Washington, DC, USA, 2016.
32. Goff, B.A.; Mandel, L.S.; Drescher, C.W.; Urban, N.; Gough, S.; Schurman, K.M.; Patras, J.; Mahony, B.S.; Andersen, M.R. Development of an ovarian cancer symptom index: Possibilities for earlier detection. *Cancer* **2007**, *109*, 221–227. [CrossRef] [PubMed]
33. Goff, B. Symptoms associated with ovarian cancer. *Clin. Obstet. Gynecol.* **2012**, *55*, 36–42. [CrossRef] [PubMed]
34. Pavlik, E.J.; Saunders, B.A.; Doran, S.; McHugh, K.W.; Ueland, F.R.; Desemone, C.P.; Depriest, P.D.; Ware, R.A.; Kryscio, R.J.; van Nagell, J.R., Jr. The search for meaning—Symptoms and transvaginal sonography screening for ovarian cancer. *Cancer* **2009**, *115*, 3689–3698. [CrossRef] [PubMed]
35. Rossing, M.A.; Wicklund, K.G.; Cushing-Haugen, K.L.; Weiss, N.S. Predictive value of symptoms for early detection of ovarian cancer. *J. Natl. Cancer Inst.* **2010**, *102*, 222–229. [CrossRef] [PubMed]
36. Cannistra, S.A. Cancer of the Ovary. *N. Engl. J. Med.* **2004**, *351*, 2519–2529. [CrossRef] [PubMed]
37. Bast, R.C.; Feeney, M.; Lazarus, H.; Nadler, L.M.; Colvin, R.B.; Knapp, R.C. Reactivity of a monoclonal antibody with human ovarian carcinoma. *J. Clin. Investig.* **1981**, *68*, 1331–1337. [CrossRef] [PubMed]
38. Gupta, D.; Lis, C.G. Role of CA125 in predicting ovarian cancer survival—A review of the epidemiological literature. *J. Ovarian Res.* **2009**, *2*, 13. [CrossRef] [PubMed]
39. Fritsche, H.A.; Bast, R.C. CA 125 in ovarian cancer: Advances and controversy. *Clin. Chem.* **1998**, *44*, 1379–1380. [PubMed]
40. Jayson, G.C.; Kohn, E.C.; Kitchener, H.C.; Ledermann, J.A. Ovarian Cancer. *Lancet* **2014**, *384*, 1376–1388. [CrossRef]
41. Moore, R.G.; Jabre-Raughley, M.; Brown, A.K.; Robison, K.M.; Miller, M.C.; Allard, W.J.; Kurman, R.J.; Bast, R.C.; Skates, S.J. Comparison of a novel multiple marker assay vs. the Risk of Malignancy Index for the prediction of epithelial ovarian cancer in patients with a pelvic mass. *Am. J. Obstet. Gynecol.* **2010**, *203*, 1–6. [CrossRef] [PubMed]
42. Novak, M.; Lukasz, J.; Stachowiak, G.; Stetkiewicz, T.; Wilczynski, J.R. Current clinical application of serum biomarkers to detect ovarian cancer. *Prz. Menopauzalny* **2015**, *14*, 254–259.
43. Thrall, M.M.; Goff, B.A.; Symons, R.G.; Flum, D.R.; Gray, H.J. Thirty-day mortality after primary cytoreductive surgery for advanced ovarian cancer in the elderly. *Obstet. Gynecol.* **2011**, *118*, 537–547. [CrossRef] [PubMed]
44. Gerestein, C.G.; Nieuwenhuyzen-de Boer, G.M.; Eijkemans, M.J.; Kooi, G.S.; Burger, C.W. Prediction of 30-day morbidity after primary cytoreductive surgery for advanced stage ovarian cancer. *Eur. J. Cancer* **2010**, *46*, 102–109. [CrossRef] [PubMed]
45. Sun, C.C.; Bodurka, D.C.; Weaver, C.B.; Rasu, R.; Wolf, J.K.; Bevers, M.W.; Smith, J.A.; Wharton, J.T.; Rubenstein, E.B. Rankings and symptom assessments of side effects from chemotherapy: Insights from experienced patients with ovarian cancer. *Support. Care Cancer* **2005**, *13*, 219–227. [CrossRef] [PubMed]
46. American Cancer Society. Chemotherapy for Ovarian Cancer. Available online: https://www.cancer.org/cancer/ovarian-cancer/treating/chemotherapy.html (accessed on 9 November 2016).

47. Guidozzi, F. Living with Ovarian Cancer. *Gynecol. Oncol.* **1992**, *50*, 202–207. [CrossRef] [PubMed]
48. Matulonis, U.A.; Kornblith, A.; Lee, H.; Bryan, J.; Gibson, C.; Wells, C.; Lee, J.; Sullivan, L.; Penson, R. Long-term adjustment of early-stage ovarian cancer survivors. *Int. J. Gynecol. Cancer* **2008**, *18*, 1183–1193. [CrossRef] [PubMed]
49. Bodurka-Bevers, D.; Basen-Engquist, K.; Carmack, C.L.; Fitzgerald, M.A.; Wolf, J.K.; de Moor, C.; Gershenson, D.M. Depression, anxiety, and quality of life in patients with epithelial ovarian cancer. *Gynecol. Oncol.* **2000**, *78*, 302–308. [CrossRef] [PubMed]
50. Butow, P.N.; Price, M.A.; Bell, M.L.; Webb, P.M.; DeFazio, A.; Australian Ovarian Cancer Study Group; Australian Ovarian Cancer Study Quality of Life Study Investigators; Friedlander, M. Caring for women with ovarian cancer in the last year of life: A longitudinal study of caregiver quality of life, distress and unmet needs. *Gynecol. Oncol.* **2014**, *132*, 690–697. [PubMed]
51. Van Nagell, J.R.; Depriest, P.D.; Gallion, H.H.; Pavlik, E.J. Ovarian cancer screening. *Cancer* **1993**, *71*, 1523–1528. [CrossRef] [PubMed]
52. Maxim, L.D.; Niebo, R.; Utell, M.J. Screening tests: A review with examples. *Inhal. Toxicol.* **2014**, *26*, 811–828. [CrossRef] [PubMed]
53. Van Nagell, J.R., Jr.; DePriest, P.D.; Ueland, F.R.; DeSimone, C.P.; Cooper, A.L.; McDonald, J.M.; Pavlik, E.J.; Kryscio, R.J. Ovarian cancer screening with annual transvaginal sonography: Findings of 25,000 women screened. *Cancer* **2007**, *109*, 1887–1896. [CrossRef] [PubMed]
54. Van Nagell, J.R.; Gallion, H.H.; Pavlik, E.J.; DePriest, P.D. Ovarian cancer screening. *Cancer* **1995**, *76*, 2086–2091. [CrossRef]
55. Pavlik, E.J.; Ueland, F.R.; Miller, R.W.; Ubellacker, J.M.; DeSimone, C.P.; Elder, J.; Hoff, J.; Baldwin, L.; Kryscio, R.J.; van Nagell, J.R., Jr. Frequency and disposition of ovarian abnormalities followed with serial transvaginal ultrasonography. *Obstet. Gynecol.* **2013**, *122*, 210–217. [CrossRef] [PubMed]
56. Van Nagell, J.R.; Hoff, J.T. Transvaginal ultrasonography in ovarian cancer screening: Current perspectives. *Int. J. Women Health* **2014**, *6*, 25–33. [CrossRef] [PubMed]
57. Elder, J.W.; Pavlik, E.J.; Long, A.; Miller, R.W.; DeSimone, C.P.; Hoff, J.T.; Ueland, W.R.; Kryscio, R.J.; van Nagell, J.R., Jr. Serial ultrasonographic evaluation of ovarian abnormalities with morphology index. *Gynecol. Oncol.* **2014**, *135*, 8–12. [CrossRef] [PubMed]
58. Buys, S.S.; Partridge, E.; Black, A.; Johnson, C.C.; Lamerato, L.; Isaacs, C.; Reding, D.J.; Greenlee, R.T.; Yokochi, L.A.; Kessel, B.; et al. Effect of screening on ovarian cancer mortality: The prostate, lung, colorectal and ovarian (PLCO) cancer screening randomized controlled trial. *JAMA* **2011**, *305*, 2295–2303. [CrossRef] [PubMed]
59. Pinsky, P.F.; Yu, K.; Kramer, B.S.; Black, A.; Buys, S.S.; Partridge, E.; Gohagan, J.; Berg, C.D. Extended mortality results for ovarian cancer screening in the PLCO trial with median 15 years follow-up. *Gynecol. Oncol.* **2016**, *135*, 270–275. [CrossRef] [PubMed]
60. Skates, S.S. OCS: Development of the Risk of Ovarian Cancer Algorithm (ROCA) and ROCA screening trials. *Int. J. Gynecol. Cancer* **2012**, *22*, S24–S26. [CrossRef] [PubMed]
61. Jacobs, I.J.; Menon, U.; Ryan, A.; Gentry-Maharaj, A.; Burnell, A.; Kalsi, J.K.; Amso, N.N.; Apostolidou, S.; Benjamin, E.; Cruickshank, D.; et al. Ovarian cancer screening and mortality in the UK collaborative trial of ovarian cancer screening (UKCTOCS): A randomized controlled trial. *Lancet* **2016**, *387*, 945–956. [CrossRef]
62. Wentzensen, N. Large ovarian cancer screening trial shows modest mortality reduction, but does not justify population-based ovarian cancer screening. *Evid. Based Med.* **2016**, *21*, 159. [CrossRef] [PubMed]
63. Kobayashi, H.; Yamada, Y.; Sado, T.; Sakata, M.; Yoshida, S.; Kawaguchi, R.; Kanayama, S.; Shigetomi, J.; Haruta, S.; Tsuji, Y.; et al. A randomized study of screening for ovarian cancer: A multicenter study in Japan. *Int. J. Gynecol. Cancer* **2008**, *18*, 414–420. [CrossRef] [PubMed]

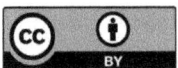

diagnostics

Review

Ultrasound Monitoring of Extant Adnexal Masses in the Era of Type 1 and Type 2 Ovarian Cancers: Lessons Learned From Ovarian Cancer Screening Trials

Eleanor L. Ormsby [1,2,*], Edward J. Pavlik [3] and John P. McGahan [1]

[1] Department of Radiology, University of California Davis Medical Center, 4860 Y Street, Suite 3100, Sacramento, CA 95817, USA; jpmcgahan@ucdavis.edu
[2] Department of Radiology, Kaiser Permanente Sacramento, 2025 Morse Ave, CA 95825, USA
[3] Division of Gynecologic Oncology, Department of Obstetrics and Gynecology, University of Kentucky Chandler Medical Center-Markey Cancer Center, Lexington, KY 40536, USA; Epaul1@uky.edu
* Correspondence: eormsby@gmail.com; Tel.: +1-917-753-3257

Academic Editor: Andreas Kjaer
Received: 9 January 2017; Accepted: 24 April 2017; Published: 28 April 2017

Abstract: Women that are positive for an ovarian abnormality in a clinical setting can have either a malignancy or a benign tumor with probability favoring the benign alternative. Accelerating the abnormality to surgery will result in a high number of unnecessary procedures that will place cost burdens on the individual and the health delivery system. Surveillance using serial ultrasonography is a reasonable alternative that can be used to discover if changes in the ovarian abnormality will occur that favor either a malignant or benign interpretation. Several ovarian cancer screening trials have had extensive experiences with changes in subclinical ovarian abnormalities in normal women that can define growth, stability or resolution and give some idea of the time frame over which changes occur. The present report examines these experiences and relates them to the current understanding of ovarian cancer ontology, presenting arguments related to the benefits of surveillance.

Keywords: ovary; cancer; screening; monitoring; surveillance; serial ultrasonography

1. Introduction

Ovarian cancer is the deadliest cancer that women face, causing more deaths than any other cancer of the female reproductive system [1]. However, the prevalence of ovarian cancer is low, responsible for only about 3% of all cancers in women [2] and accounting for a lifetime risk of 1.3% (1 in 75) [3]. Transvaginal ultrasound (TVS) has been widely recognized as the first line for evaluating adnexal masses presenting both low risk and low cost. Prospective ovarian cancer screening trials have utilized TVS to detect early stage malignancies. The five-year survival rate for women diagnosed with stage I ovarian cancer has been reported to be as high as 95% [4,5] in contrast to only 30% for women with stage III disease [6]. While large prospective screening trials have focused on how best to identify malignancies in asymptomatic women in the general population, adnexal masses are commonly identified by ultrasound ordered for a wide variety of indications in routine clinical practice even when a patient does not present with relevant symptoms. While the US Preventive Services Task Force (USPSTF) has recommended against population screening for ovarian cancer [7], many women undergo ultrasound for various symptoms. This paper reviews recent prospective ovarian cancer screening trial findings for clinical application on how women with adnexal masses, found by ultrasound, for various reasons other than for screening purposes, should be managed and followed.

Ovarian cysts are often observed sonographically even in post-menopausal women with a reported incidence rate of up to 21% [8]. The question of how best to manage these masses has been the subject of much interest and debate among clinicians including obstetric gynecologists, primary care physicians, radiologists and gynecology oncologists. Several reports have asserted that resected ovarian cysts do not contain malignancy [9–11], but that if left unmonitored, ovarian cysts can progress to ovarian cancers [12,13]. Therefore, all ovarian cysts may present some source of concern. Historically, this concern has led to a conundrum among radiologists and clinicians. Should these cysts be monitored (how frequently and for how long) or should ovarian cysts be managed operatively at the risk of potential harm from surgical complications and medical expenses?

In 2010, a consensus panel of the Society of Radiologists in Ultrasound (SRU) that was composed of 19 experts in radiology, obstetric gynecology, and gynecology oncology, as well as pathology released a recommendation regarding the management of adnexal masses found sonographically in asymptomatic women [14]. The panel analyzed literature available at the time of the conference (October 2009) and strategies in clinical practice with the goal of reaching a consensus on: (1) which masses might not require follow-up, (2) which masses would need imaging follow-up, as well as when follow-up evaluation should occur, and (3) which masses should warrant referral to a gynecologic oncologist for surgical evaluation. The consensus agreed that it is reasonable to perform annual ultrasound follow-up of cysts larger than 5 cm in premenopausal women and those larger than 1 cm in postmenopausal women, although such cysts are unlikely to be malignant [14]. A recent expert review suggested that low risk abnormalities can undergo an initial three-month follow-up with those that remain stable or decreasing in size being examined every 12 months for five years [15].

Since the SRU guidelines from 2010 [14], differences over how best to manage adnexal masses persisted and were recently addressed by the first international consensus conference on adnexal masses [15]. This panel included representatives of societies in the fields of gynecology, gynecologic oncology, radiology and pathology and clinicians from Europe, Canada and the United States. While many of the adnexal masses are benign appearing (i.e., simple cysts or hemorrhagic cysts), for many more, it is not clear whether the mass may contain foci of malignancy and consequently are classified as *indeterminate*. As a clarification of terminology, "simple cysts" and "unilocular cysts" are the same and are characterized as being anechoic structures that are absent papillae, solid areas and septa (complete or incomplete). The low prevalence of ovarian cancer (3%) [2] establishes the likelihood that most ovarian cysts are benign yet cysts cannot be dismissed because they occur with a high incidence rate (21–35%) [8]. Some cysts are not simple and include morphologic elements that can demonstrate multiseptations or small solid nodules. No specific guideline had been established for indeterminate masses by the SRU consensus due to the fact that data analyzing long-term follow up of adnexal masses at the time was insufficient. The SRU stated that "as research continues, the recommendations regarding management of adnexal cysts may vary". The present review examines the evidence from recent research in histopathology of ovarian cancer types, ovarian cancer screening trials and ultrasound morphology of adnexal masses to establish a framework for surveillance of these masses.

2. Type 1 and Type 2 Ovarian Cancers Found in Ultrasound Imaging

Currently, ovarian cancers now include two distinct types of malignancy: Type 1 or 2 based on histologic pathogenesis, molecular alterations and clinical progression (Table 1). Type 1 ovarian cancers include low grade serous carcinoma, endometrioid carcinoma, and clear cell carcinoma. Type 1 ovarian cancers demonstrate a step-wise progression originating from a benign precursor or borderline tumor or endometriosis [16–18]. For example, low grade serous carcinomas may arise via transformation of benign and borderline serous tumors that are thought to be derived from inclusion cysts originating from the ovarian surface or tubal epithelium. This progression is analogous to the adenoma-to-carcinoma sequence seen in colorectal carcinoma pathogenesis or the hyperplasia-to-carcinoma sequence in endometrioid carcinoma of the endometrium [19].

In contrast, Type 2 ovarian cancers are highly aggressive and include high grade serous, high grade endometrioid and undifferentiated carcinomas, as well as malignant mixed mesodermal carcinomas, usually presenting at an advanced stage [17,19,20]. Type 2 ovarian cancers often have TP53 mutations but rarely have mutations that are associated with Type 1 ovarian malignancies [17,20]. Some Type 2 ovarian cancers (in particular, high grade serous carcinoma) are associated with *BRCA* (BReast CAncer susceptibility gene) inactivation [21]. Compelling evidence indicates that these malignancies may originate from the epithelium of the fimbrial portion of the fallopian tube as serous tubal intraepithelial carcinomas (STIC) [22–32]. Finally, some high grade serous carcinomas have been reported to develop from transformation of serous borderline tumors or low grade Type 1 serous carcinomas [17–20]. While pathogenesis may differ, the morphology of the high-grade serous carcinomas that develop in the Type 2 pathway is similar to high-grade serous carcinomas that are transformed from Type 1 tumors with shared clinical behaviors [17]. Using this paradigm, a stratified treatment plan can be devised. However, currently there is no prospective means that differentiates between the subtypes of ovarian cancer based on ultrasound imaging. Based on recent ovarian cancer screening results, abnormalities with lesser degrees of morphologic complexity may harbor micro foci of ovarian cancer indicating that a wide spectrum of abnormal morphology should be considered for ultrasound follow up and active surveillance.

Table 1. Summary of Type 1 and Type 2 ovarian carcinomas.

Tumor Type	Type 1 Tumors	Type 2 Tumors
Behavior	Indolent	Aggressive
Diagnosis at	Early Stage	Advanced Stage
Survival Rate at 5 years	About 55%	About 30%
Type/Precursor	-Endometrioid carcinoma/Endometriosis -Clear cell carcinoma/Endometriosis Mucinous carcinoma/Mucinous Cystadenoma, Endometriosis, Teratoma, -Brenner Tumor, and Mucinous borderline tumor -Low grade serous carcinoma/Serous cystadenoma, Adenofibroma, Atypical proliferative serous tumor, Mullerian epithelial cyst -Transitional cell carcinoma or Malignant Brenner tumor/ Brenner tumor	-High grade serous carcinoma/Probably de novo starting at the tubo, ovarian surface epithelium, serous tubal intraepithelial carcinomas (STIC) or ovarian hilum stem cell -Undifferentiated carcinoma? -Malignant mixed carcinoma?

2.1. Summary of Information from Recent Prospective Ovarian Cancer Screening Trials

There have been four large prospective ovarian cancer screening trials utilizing ultrasound in asymptomatic women [5,33–35]. The first randomized control trial in the US was the Prostate, Lung, Colorectal and Ovarian Cancer Screening (PLCO) Trial, a randomized controlled trial (RCT) of 68,616 women aged 55 to 74 of whom 30,630 underwent screening between 1993 and 2007 [34]. Women were screened using serum CA-125 (cancer antigen 125) at a cut-off of $\geq$35 kU/L and transvaginal ultrasound (TVS) for four years followed by CA-125 alone for an additional two years. Endpoint analysis showed that screening with the combination of CA-125 and transvaginal ultrasound had no mortality benefit compared to the unscreened control group [34]. Importantly, in the PLCO study, surgical decisions were made on the basis of a single ultrasound exam and an absolute CA-125 level of 35 units/mL. More importantly, the PLCO trial had no uniform evaluation and treatment algorithm for patients with screen-detected adnexal masses so that women identified in the screening arm could be treated up to nine months after ultrasound detection, allowing their disease to progress to later stages during this time.

In the multicenter prospective randomized Shizuoka Cohort Study of Ovarian Cancer Screening (SCSOCS) trial in Japan [33], conducted between 1985 and 1999, asymptomatic postmenopausal women were assigned either to a screening arm (n = 41,688) or to a control arm (n = 40,799). Furthermore,

63% of ovarian cancers detected by screening were stage I disease versus 38% in the control arm. Importantly, optimal tumor debulking was achieved more often in women whose ovarian cancer was detected by screening [33]. Assessment of ovarian cancer specific survival was not completed in the SCSOCS trial.

More recent studies have been published with a screening strategy that improves on using a single ultrasound exam or a single CA-125 value at 35 units/mL, an approach that did not achieve an acceptable positive predictive value (PPV) in the PLCO trial [34]. These strategies include the use of serial ultrasound instead of a single ultrasound exam dictating the surgical decision and the utilization of multimodalities keying on changes in serial CA 125 determinations. The University of Kentucky Ovarian Cancer Screening Trial utilized a prospective single arm that focused on annual ultrasound screening study of 25,327 women from 1987 to 2012 [36]. In the Kentucky study, serial ultrasound follow up of the 6807 women with ovarian abnormalities displaying varying ultrasonographic morphologic features resulted in a 304% improved PPV from 8.1% to 25% and reduced unnecessary surgery on benign tumors [36]. Importantly, this study found that women in the screening group had a higher rate of earlier stage cancer discovery (68% stage I or II disease) than the unscreened comparison group (27% stage I or II, $p < 0.01$) [36–38]. Overall five-year survival of women who had epithelial ovarian cancer (EOC) found during the serial ultrasound follow up including false negative cancers was 74.8% ± 6.6% compared to 53.7% ± 2.3% for women who were clinically detected ($p < 0.01$) [37,38]. Using the serial ultrasound approach, differentiating benign from malignant tumors was based on the regression of benign masses [36]. Extending serial ultrasound to include a quantitative index showed that malignant tumors demonstrated increasing morphology index scores over time [37,39].

Others have evaluated serial CA-125 level or other biomarkers such as human epididymis protein 4 (HE4) to improve the detection of ovarian cancer [40–42]. The Risk of Ovarian Cancer Algorithm (ROCA) is a multivariate linear model based on longitudinal data from women with ovarian cancer and estimates intermediate and high risk for malignancy based on changes in CA-125 levels relative to an individual's previous levels. ROCA with multiple CA-125 determinations has performed better in detecting ovarian cancer than a single level since CA-125 levels vary greatly depending on the menopausal status, fertility drug use, current cigarette use, race, pelvic inflammation and irregular menstruation [43]. Using an absolute CA-125 cut off value of 35 units/mL may result in a high false negative rate because only 50–60% of women with stage 1 EOC will have CA-125 elevated above this level and borderline, and Type 1 or low grade tumors are known to express low levels of CA-125 [44].

In the United Kingdom Collaborative Trial of Ovarian Cancer Screening (UKCTOC), the largest randomized control screening trial to date, performed between 2001–2005, 202,638 women from the general population were assigned to a control group (no intervention) or to annual screening using either transvaginal ultrasound (USS) or serum CA-125 interpreted by ROCA with transvaginal ultrasound as a second line test (multimodal screening, MMS) [12,35,44]. The stage distribution of the screen-detected primary invasive cancers was similar in both the multimodality group and the group that received only ultrasonography [35]. In addition, 50% of primary invasive ovarian and tubal malignancies detected by serial ultrasound screening alone had stage I or II disease versus 26% in the control cases detected clinically (i.e., without screening) [35]. Screening produced a significant increase in the detection of early stage ovarian malignancy. A report on the survival benefit from the UKCTOCS has been published, which showed that, when prevalent cases were excluded, a significant mortality reduction was noted after 7–14 years within the multimodality arm [35]. Similar but lesser mortality reduction was seen with ultrasound alone. The trial is currently undergoing additional follow up to further examine mortality reduction. Based on these data, it was concluded that 641 screens are needed to prevent one ovarian cancer death [35].

Recently, it has been reported that ovarian cancer screening detects more indolent and less aggressive Type 1 cancers [45] and that the frequency of Type 2 cancer is ~75% is higher than Type 1 with higher mortality rate for Type 2 cancer due to its faster rate of growth and metastasis. This result is in contrast to findings from the Kentucky Ovarian Cancer Screening trial where 83.3% of early stage malignancies were aggressive Type 2 cancers [5,35,36,38]. In the UKCTOC ultrasound arm trial, both Type 1 and Type 2 cancers were detected albeit more Type 1 than Type 2 [35]. Of the 23 Type 2 cancers diagnosed in the UKCTOC ultrasound arm, 15 were associated with adnexal abnormalities, while eight had normal ultrasound with subsequent diagnosis of ovarian cancer within 16 months (ranging 6–13 months with median of 10) [12]. No women with persisting normal ultrasound results were found to have Type 1 ovarian cancers of the 32 women with Type 1 cancer who were detected by ultrasound in the ultrasound arm of the UKCTOC [12]. Based on these observations, it may be concluded that many Type 2 cancers are found in women brought to clinical practice by symptoms and that Type 2 cancers have been shown to be quite possible to find through ovarian cancer screening using ultrasonography. Therefore, serial ultrasound follow up of persistent masses may benefit women in clinical practice by discriminating lethal Type 2 ovarian cancers as well as by reducing unnecessary surgery in cases where complexity moderates or abnormalities resolve.

2.2. Can Type 2 Ovarian Cancers Be Detected by Ultrasound?

Using a growth model of serous cystadenocarcinoma (Type 2) based on retrospective analysis of $BRCA_1$ carriers who had undergone prophylactic bilateral salpingo-oophorectomies (PBSOs), it was noted that high grade serous carcinoma likely spends approximately 4.3 years as histopathologically detectable but clinically occult early stage tumors [46]. This analysis also stated that more than 50% of serous carcinomas advanced to stage III/IV by the time they reached 3 cm in diameter. Assuming spherical shape, this would be a volume of 14 cm^3 (note that the normal ovary is 10–20 cm^3 and a walnut is 22 cm^3). The report postulated that the tumor would double in volume every two and a half months so that, at best, ultrasound follow up may only lead to the detection of low volume high grade Type 2 cancers rather than early stage cases. However, early stage disease detected in the Kentucky Ovarian Screening Program was larger than postulated by this model (Stage I Type 2: 65.4 cm^3 ± 27.6, 27, 4.1, 366, n = 13; Stage II Type 2: 131.1 cm^3 ± 33.4, 95.8, 10, 351.4, n = 14 (mean ± SEM, median, min, max)) [5,37]. Thus, the prediction made by the model [46] that to achieve 50% sensitivity in detecting tumors before they advance to Stage III, an annual screen would need to detect tumors of 1.3 cm in diameter is inaccurate and not supported by empirical screening data. Other investigators modeling the levels of CA-125 associated with the smallest progressing ovarian cancers reported that these cancers could develop unnoticed for 10.1 years and presented the view that the largest tumor below the resolution of ultrasound (0.5 cm diameter) could progress to a detectable size (1.2–2.5 cm) in 1–2 years [47]. Based on this estimation [47] and the Kentucky findings summarized above, early stage Type 2 ovarian malignancies are well within the range of discovery by ultrasound. In the context of surveillance monitoring, it would seem that arbitrary cessation as suggested by one retrospective study [48] of ultrasound follow up of small complex adnexal masses, which are less than 6 cm at seven months would miss both small volume high grade Type 2 cancers and the indolent Type 1 tumors that can potentially progress to higher grade invasive cancer.

3. Risk of Ovarian Cancer When There Is an Adnexal Mass

Adapting the information from these prospective ovarian cancer screening trials to non-screening applications in day-to-day clinical practice needs consideration. The USPSTF has recommended against ultrasound exams for ovarian cancer screen in asymptomatic women [7] based on prior randomized prospective ovarian cancer trials that failed to show mortality benefits while focusing on the risk of unnecessary surgery with a small immediate complication rate or more long-term effects of premature menopause from oophorectomy such as bone density loss. However, women present clinically with a wide variety of indications including nonspecific symptoms, as well as more gynecologic symptoms such as vaginal bleeding, pelvic fullness or pain. Sometimes, women may be referred for follow up ultrasound on incidental abnormal findings from other diagnostic radiology exams such as CT that have been obtained for unrelated reasons. Women who had any adnexal mass had a much higher relative risk of developing ovarian cancer as observed in the UKCTOC trial, compared to women who had no adnexal mass [12]. The relative risk ratio for all EOC (Types 1 and 2) was 49.2 for women with a multilocular solid cyst and 38.4 for women with a solid mass when compared to women with normal ultrasound exams [12]. For the most deadly and aggressive ovarian cancers (Type 2), the relative risk was 31.3 for women with a multilocular cysts with solid components and 38.4 for women with a solid mass [12].

Even benign appearing unilocular and multilocular cysts without any solid elements have been reported to be associated with epithelial ovarian cancer. In the UKCTOC report, unilocular and multilocular cysts without any solid components had a relative risk for EOC within three years of 5.3 (95% CI (confidence interval) 1.9–15.2) and 6.8 (95% CI 1.9–22.9), respectively, compared to normal ultrasound exams [12]. Among the primary EOC detected in the UKCTOC ultrasound screening trial, 16% (nine out of 55) developed from unilocular cysts while 9% (five out of 55) developed from multilocular cysts within three years of an initial scan. Among the borderline tumor and Type 1 epithelial cancers, 16% (five out of 32) developed from unilocular cysts while 13% (four out of 32) developed from multilocular cysts [12]. In another series by a separate research group, 11% (4/35) of borderline tumors and 4% (1/24) of epithelial ovarian cancers were classified as unilocular cysts at ultrasound examination performed by an ultrasound expert in a tertiary referral center for gynecological ultrasound [49].

Valentin et al. noted in their cohort that the overall malignancy rate for unilocular cysts was 1% and was higher among postmenopausal women (2.76%) then premenopausal women (0.54%) [50]. While the rates were very low, the difference was statistically significant between the two age groups. The authors of the study noted that, upon pathologic inspection, seven of the 11 malignant cysts described as unilocular on ultrasounds were found to contain small papillary projections or solid components, which were not observed sonographically [50]. Careful scrutiny of ultrasound images was advocated because subjective error or ultrasound resolution may provide explanations for the failure to observe the papillary projections. While there are limitations to ultrasound, the degree to which these limitations contribute to ultrasound results is small as shown by high sensitivities ($\geq$80%) and high negative predictive values (>99%) [5,37,38].

3.1. The Risk Profile for Abnormal Ultrasound Findings

Among postmenopausal women in the general US population, the overall risk of ovarian cancer rises with age to a 9–13% lifetime risk [51]. Relative risk increases when symptoms are present for which a pelvic ultrasound is often performed in clinical practice, mostly because of pelvic pain. The great majority of women with symptoms alone do not have an ovarian malignancy. The majority of women with both symptoms and an ovarian abnormality on ultrasound also do not have a malignancy due to the low prevalence of ovarian cancer; however, women with symptoms have been found to have a higher prevalence of ovarian cancer than that reported for asymptomatic women in screening trials using ultrasonography [52–54]. Differences between screening trial pelvic ultrasound outcomes and those in clinical settings result because symptoms predominate in clinical settings.

3.2. Benefit of Serial Ultrasound Follow-Up

Serial ultrasound and a subsequent increase in morphologic complexity of an adnexal mass have been used as the basis for surgical decisions in the single arm trial at the University of Kentucky [37] and in the UKCTOC [35]. In the University of Kentucky trial, the majority of ovarian abnormalities resolved within a year with serial ultrasound, including indeterminate masses. More than half of women (63%) with ovarian cystic abnormalities had resolution in the subsequent follow-up with near exponential resolution of ovarian abnormalities so that, by 1–2 years, only a fraction of the ovarian abnormalities persisted (Figure 1, from [36]).

Ovarian abnormalities that continue to persist comprise only a fraction of the ovarian abnormalities that are identified and are candidates for ongoing serial observation until their indeterminate status changes due to an increase in morphologic complexity. Therefore, serial ultrasound surveillance can mitigate the potential risk from surgical complications due to prematurely resecting indeterminate adnexal masses, especially if an adnexal mass demonstrates signs of resolving. Ultrasound follow-up is advantageous because it is cost effective and low risk. The cost of ultrasound follow-up is nominal compared to the cost of surgical treatment for women [55] and provides a greater margin of safety than dismissing an extant adnexal mass without follow-up based on presuming benign status due to an initial indeterminate ultrasound morphology.

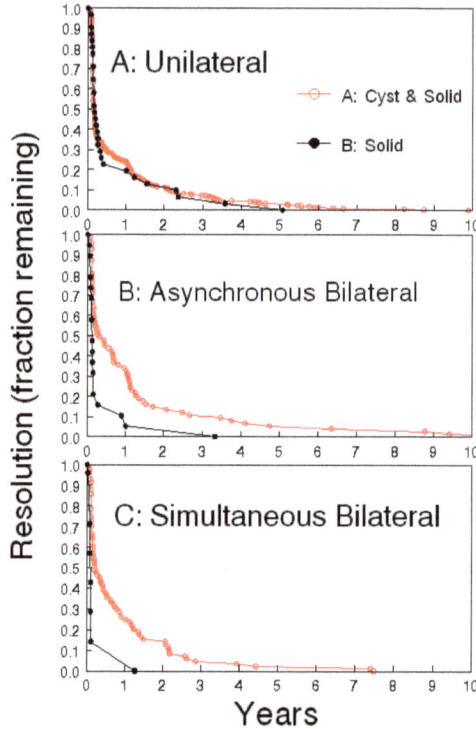

Figure 1. Resolution of complex ovarian abnormalities. (**A**) unilateral abnormalities, never simultaneously on both sides; (**B**) intermittent unilateral abnormalities consisting of ovarian abnormality on one side or the other at different times; (**C**) bilateral abnormalities occurring simultaneously on both sides. Cysts with solid components: red open circles. Solid components: black solid circles. Intrapanel comparisons, (**A**): not statistically different. (**B**) $p < 0.001$, (**C**) $p < 0.001$. Interpanel comparisons: **A** vs. **C** $p < 0.01$, **A** vs. **B** and **B** vs. **C**, not significantly different.

4. Subjectivity

4.1. Does Stability Over Time Argue Against Malignancy?

To address this question, work that focused on the ultrasound discovery of adnexal masses was reviewed [13]. Malignancy has been found in stable masses, which enlarged and increased in morphologic complexity in up to three years after initial detection in the UKCTOCS [12]. To put the risk of prematurely terminating ultrasound surveillance in perspective, the definition of the acceptable risk level (ARL) from environmental studies [56] of no more than 1 extra death/100,000 was used to normalize the UKCTOCS trial data. Using this approach, the absolute risks for the appearance of malignancy in up to three years after an initial ultrasound exam as calculated from the UKCTOCS data [12] are considerably elevated (Figure 2). The risk of malignancy is higher after finding any of the ovarian ultrasound abnormalities as judged by the 95% CI (Figure 2). Even allowing the 0.001% ARL to be relaxed 10 fold would still lead to the expectation of a considerable number of extra malignancies within three years of the first scan. If prematurely stopping surveillance caused 50% or more of these malignancies to be diagnosed at an advanced stage, likely destined to be fatal, then extra deaths due to curtailing surveillance can be expected to be high and emphasizes the peril of limiting ultrasound surveillance [13].

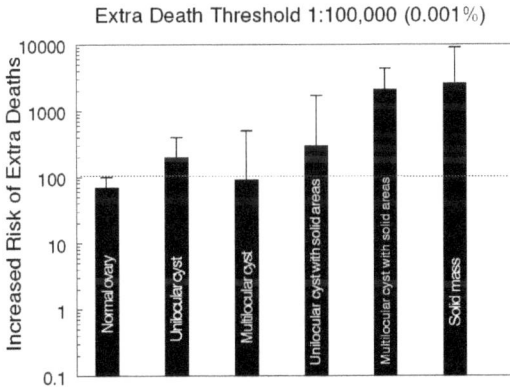

Figure 2. Estimation of risk in terms of extra deaths in women diagnosed with Type 2 primary epithelial ovarian cancer within three years after an ultrasound exam. Data were collected in the United Kingdom Collaborative Trial of Ovarian Cancer Screening Protocols as published [12] and normalized by the acceptable level of risk of no more than one extra death per 100,000 in environmental studies. Absolute risk of subsequent malignancy is shown by the bar labeled with each type of finding on the first ultrasound exam. The 95% confidence interval extends upward from each bar. The dashed line indicates the 95% confidence interval of the normal ovary extended across all types of findings.

4.2. The Conundrum of Ultrasound: Subjectivity and Technical Considerations

Subjectivity and operator-dependent errors are intrinsic to ultrasound imaging even when the images are acquired and interpreted by expert radiologists or gynecologists and contain subtle features that can go unreported or be missed. While the term *expert sonographer* is in wide use, there is no definition that provides an understanding of this status or terminology. Ultrasounds are very often performed by technologists whose varying skills and expertise are acquired and honed in the practice in which they are employed. For experts and technologists alike, small lesions can be missed due to various technical factors such as subject motion, lack of patient cooperation, large body habitus with poor acoustic penetration, bowel gas shadowing which obscures pelvic organs, positioning of the ovarian structure behind the uterus, etc. For some large masses, complete visualization of the wall and internal morphology cannot be obtained because the signal from the transvaginal probe cannot adequately reach the entire mass. When this is the case, the SRU recommendations advocate pelvic magnetic resonance images (MRIs) for better characterization and full visualization of large masses [14]. Small papillary projections within unilocular cysts can be absent on ultrasound, but later confirmed by surgical pathology. Thus, there can be situations where information from ultrasound can be inadequate.

Although ultrasound is highly sensitive, subjectivity inherent to the interpretation of ultrasound images accounts for variation in ultrasound reports especially for indeterminate adnexal masses. Recently, the International Ovarian Tumor Analysis (IOTA) study showed that there is considerable uncertainly and inter-observer disagreement when solid components and papillary projection were present [57]. Most disagreement was on the definition of a papillary projection, but there was also uncertainty leading to disagreement about whether a certain structure should be classified as a solid component or as a collection of septa, a collection of small cysts or as ovarian stroma. Including Doppler imaging can introduce variability because some septa can only be visualized with Doppler and, therefore it can change the type of morphology that is reported.

In addition to physiological cysts, serous and mucinous cystadenomas, transitional and germ cell tumors, struma ovarii, stromal cell tumors, fibromas, endometriomas, low malignant potential (borderline) tumors, and malignancies, and other structures that are expected to have the potential to be reported as having solid components in ultrasound exams of the adnexa include: inflammations, infections and abscesses. Only after surgery has been performed is it possible to establish the histopathologic identity of an ovarian abnormality seen on ultrasound. Histopathological identification is not a possibility in serial ultrasound surveillance when solid structures resolve as has been reported in the Kentucky study [36]. In brief, this study reported that while cysts with solid components had the highest risk for epithelial ovarian cancer, many complex abnormalities (cysts with apparent solid areas) and apparent solid masses were more likely to resolve within a year of surveillance (76.5–80.6%) than unilocular cysts and cysts with septations (32.8–43.9%, $p < 0.001$) [36]. Complex abnormalities and solid masses had a median time to resolution of 7.8–8.7 weeks, while unilocular cysts and cysts with septations had a median time to resolution of 53–55.6 weeks. The expectation is that if these were truly solid masses that are highly suspicious for cancer, they should not resolve. There are several possibilities to explain this observation. First, something other than the ovary was measured in the ultrasound report (i.e., overlapping adjacent tissue like a bowel loop). Second, the plane through which a partially solid ovarian structure was sonographically examined exaggerated the extent to which the structure appeared to be solid. Third, unverified factors like inflammation, infection or abscess were responsible for reporting solid areas in the ultrasound report, providing pseudo-findings. Serial ultrasonography provides a protection against a pseudo-finding of solid structure whenever there is evidence of a resolving process or resolution. Few would argue that uncertainty can be eliminated in ultrasound exams, especially with subjective interpretation providing the foundation for what is reported. The degree to which subjective interpretation can account for the identification of apparently "solid components" that subsequently resolve is not presently known, but can be corrected by a serial ultrasound imaging approach in diagnostic imaging. Moreover, the utilization of complementary Doppler imaging could contribute to differentiating a truly solid mass as distinct from a mass of clotted blood. However, even with Doppler imaging, not all solid masses will be able to demonstrate Doppler flow if there is too much tissue for the ultrasound beam to penetrate or if certain tumors are not sufficiently vascularized for detection by Doppler imaging. Thus, in the absence of definitive Doppler identification, the best solution for distinguishing apparently solid components is serial ultrasonography.

5. Ovarian Mass Ultrasound Morphology

There is considerable overlap between the ultrasonographic morphology of ovarian masses. In the UKCTOCS study, 25 (78.1%) of the borderline/Type 1 cancers had adnexal abnormalities with solid elements (unilocular solid/multilocular solid cysts or solid masses) on the initial ($n = 23$) or subsequent ($n = 2$) scans [12]. Of the 23 women diagnosed with Type 2 EOC, 15 had sonographic adnexal abnormalities where eleven (47.8%) had solid elements or ascites on the initial scan [12]. While in the UKCTOCS study, the strongest association between ovarian morphology and epithelial ovarian cancer was the presence of "solid component(s)", borderline, and Type 1 and Type 2 cancers were found across all sonographic morphologies including unilocular and multilocular cysts without solid components. In contrast, benign pathology was the norm for all morphologies including cysts with solid components [36]. The challenge for radiologists and gynecologic oncologists is correctly diagnosing epithelial ovarian cancers associated with indeterminate masses having multiple thick septations and or solid components that can be seen across borderline, indolent Type 1 tumors, aggressive Type 2 tumors and benign masses. This challenge is complicated by the low prevalence of ovarian cancer. Clear expressions of ovarian abnormalities seen ultrasonographically are presented in Figure 3. Tumors of low malignant potential (i.e., borderline tumors) account for 15% of all epithelial ovarian cancers (Figure 3A). Nearly 75% of these tumors are stage I at the time of diagnosis. They represent a heterogeneous group and occur in younger women with favorable prognosis. However, symptomatic recurrence and death may be found as long as 20 years after therapy in some patients. While low grade serous tumors (Type 1) occur less frequently, pernicious high-grade serous carcinomas (Type 2) predominate, accounting for over half of ovarian malignancies, Figure 3B. Undifferentiated carcinomas (Figure 3C, 2%), malignant mixed mesodermal tumors (Figure 3D, 3%) and high grade transitional cell carcinomas (Figure 3E, 2%) (all Type 2) each carry a serious prognosis, but together account for less than 10% of ovarian malignancies. Endometriod carcinomas comprise ~20% of ovarian malignancies with low and high grade endometriod carcinomas appearing ultrasonographically similar (Figure 3F,G). Together with clear cell carcinomas (Figure 3H, 3%), malignant Brenner's tumor (Figure 3I, <1%) and mucinous carcinomas (Figure 3J,K, 5%) are recognized as being responsive to treatment. Overlapping morphological components characterize all of these tumors. To discriminate malignant from benign abnormalities, a Morphology Index (MI) has been developed at the University of Kentucky [58]. The MI grades an abnormality on the basis of both size and structure (morphology) as shown in Figure 4. Increasing MI scores correlate well with the risk of an abnormality being malignant [39].

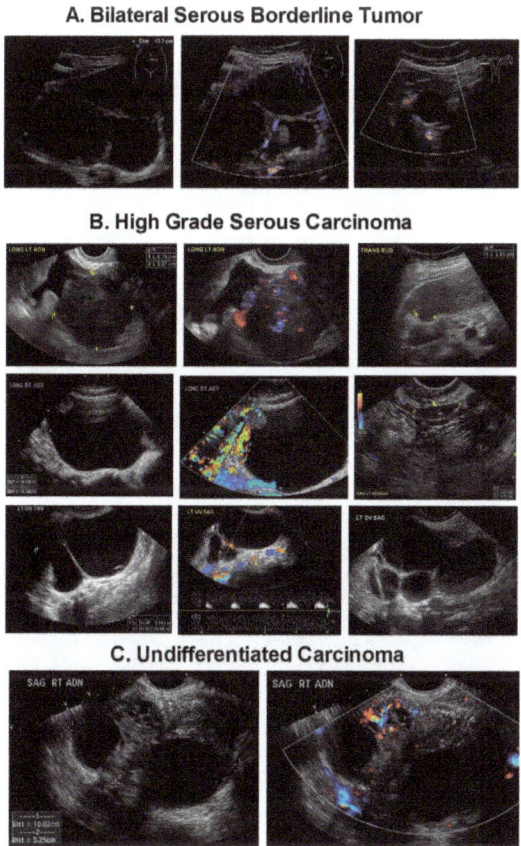

A. Bilateral Serous Borderline Tumor

B. High Grade Serous Carcinoma

C. Undifferentiated Carcinoma

Figure 3. *Cont.*

D. Malignant Mixed Mesodermal Tumor

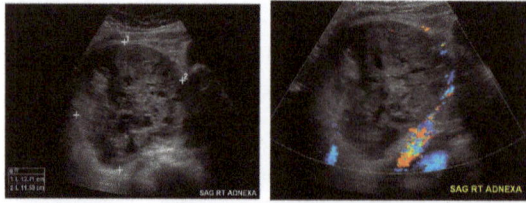

E. High Grade Transitional Cell Carcinoma

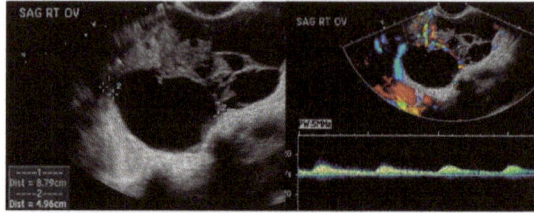

F. Low Grade Endometriod Carcinoma

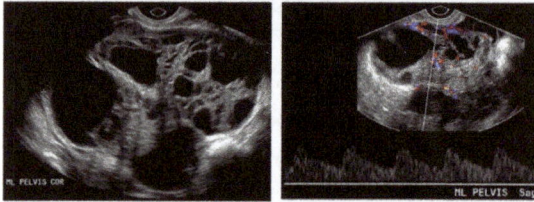

G. High Grade Endometriod Carcinoma

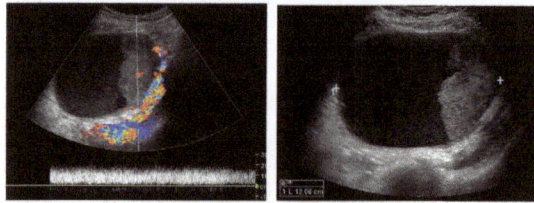

H. Clear Cell Carcinoma

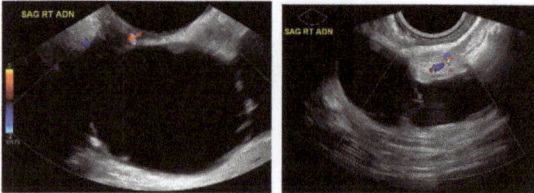

I. Malignant Brenner Tumor

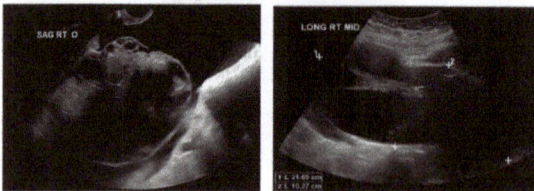

Figure 3. *Cont.*

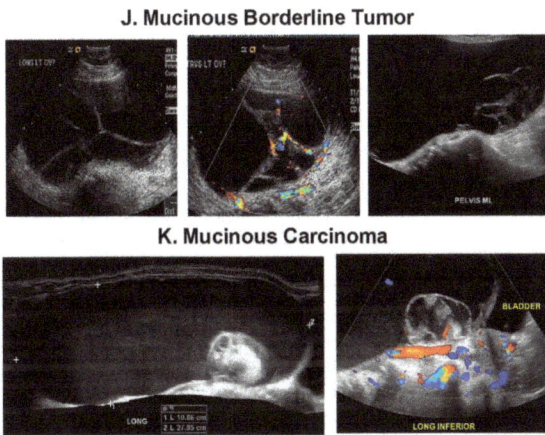

J. Mucinous Borderline Tumor

K. Mucinous Carcinoma

Figure 3. Ultrasonographic appearance of borderline, Type 1 and Type 2 ovarian cancers. (**A**) Bilateral Serous Borderline Tumor: tumors of low malignant potential (i.e., borderline tumors) account for 15% of all epithelial ovarian cancers. Nearly 75% of these tumors are stage I at the time of diagnosis. They represent a heterogeneous group and occur in younger women with favorable prognosis. However, symptomatic recurrence and death may be found as long as 20 years after therapy in some patients. (**B**) High Grade Serous Carcinoma (Type 2): serous carcinomas comprise the majority of ovarian carcinomas. Unlike low-grade serous carcinoma, *TP53* mutation occurs in up to 80% of high-grade tumors [17,20]. (**C**) Undifferentiated Carcinoma (Type 2): about 5% of ovarian cancers are so poorly differentiated and difficult to classify that they are called undifferentiated carcinomas and occur as large, solid hemorrhagic structures with necrosis. (**D**) Malignant Mixed Mesodermal Tumor (Type 2): occur almost exclusively in postmenopausal women. (**E**) High grade transitional cell carcinoma (Type 2) is probably not a distinct entity but a poorly differentiated form of serous or endometrioid carcinoma. (**F**) Low Grade Endometrioid Carcinoma (Type 1): endometriosis a likely precursor of endometrioid carcinoma. (**G**) High grade Endometriod carcinoma (Type 2) is morphologically indistinguishable from high grade serous carcinoma. (**H**) Clear Cell Carcinoma (Type 1): as with endometrioid carcinomas, there is a close association between endometriosis and clear cell carcinoma. (**I**) Malignant Brenner Tumor (Type 1): relatively uncommon neoplasm. Most Brenner tumors are benign, only 2–5% being malignant. (**J**) Mucinous Borderline Tumor (Type 1): 53.3% of borderline tumors are serous tumors and 42.5% are mucinous tumors (42.5%). (**K**) Mucinous Carcinoma (Type 1): frequently has a heterogeneous composition with coexisting elements of cystadenoma, stromal microinvasion, noninvasive carcinoma, and invasive carcinoma.

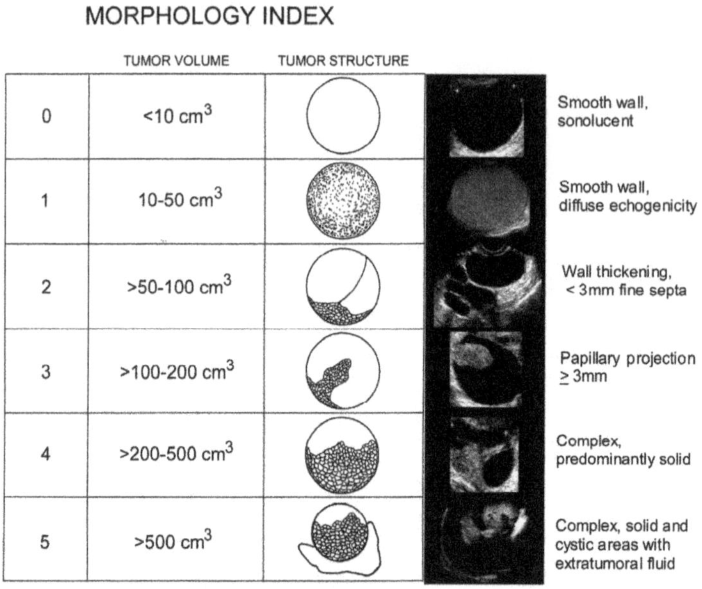

MORPHOLOGY INDEX

Figure 4. Morphology Index evaluation of ovarian abnormalities. Part of the figure is reprinted from [39,58].

5.1. Malignant Degeneration of Benign Masses

It is well known that epithelial ovarian carcinomas can develop from ovarian endometriosis [59–63]. The strongest association is seen with endometrioid and clear cell carcinomas [64–66], which have been reported to be associated with ovarian endometriosis in 30–40% and 40–70% of cases, respectively [66,67]. Endometrioid cancer is considered as a Type 1 tumor while clear cell carcinoma is a more intermediate type [16]. Twenty-eight per cent of benign and 38% of borderline endometrioid tumors were reported to be associated with endometriosis in one series [68,69]. Thus, there are benign entities that can become malignant.

5.2. Psychosocial Elements in Prospective Ovarian Cancer Screening Trials

In an age when patients can freely review their medical charts, including their entire radiology report, and access the Internet for information, we enter uncharted territory in how to communicate our findings with patients. The cost in following an ovarian mass by ultrasound is nominal compared to surgery or extensive chemo-radiation treatment when ovarian cancer is detected at a later stage. When women were polled about screening for ovarian cancer by the University of Kentucky Ovarian Cancer trial team, 97% of the women surveyed reported that they wanted to be screened and that they would even pay for screening themselves because ovarian cancer has a mortality ratio that is four times greater than breast cancer, despite an incidence rate that is low [70] even with potential complications that range from long-term physiological changes such as bone density loss to surgical mortality.

It is legitimate to consider if serial ultrasound and surveillance impacts psychosocial well-being. Non-physical or psychological harm to women has been examined in the Kentucky Ovarian Screening trial. When compared to an age and education matched group with no history of ovarian screening, women in the Kentucky trial had more ovarian cancer-specific distress/anxiety, less optimism, and less knowledge about risk factors upon entry [71]. Thus, some distress or anxiety relative to ovarian cancer appears to play a motivating role for entering the Kentucky screening trial. As part of these efforts, the validity of self-reporting by women in the Kentucky trial was evaluated and found to be very high [72]. In a study with baseline, two-week and four-month measurement, recipients of a normal ovarian screening exam showed decreased ovarian cancer-related distress, increased positive effects and increased knowledge of risk factors [73], indicating, for the vast majority of women screened, that there are beneficial effects on ovarian cancer-specific anxiety, attitude and knowledge. Women who received an abnormal TVS screening result were found to have an elevated ovarian cancer-specific distress (but not general distress) at a two-week follow-up that returned to baseline at the four-month follow-up [74]. Results were influenced by a monitoring coping style, low optimism and family history of ovarian cancer. Needs that have been identified in women with an abnormal TVS screening result deal with anticipation, emotional responses, role of the sonographer and impact of prior cancer experiences [75]. In examining social cognitive processing vs. cognitive social health processing after an abnormal TVS screening, analyses found that greater distress was associated with greater social constraint [76]. Thus, psychological conditions that are apparently associated with ovarian screening are governed by different underlying factors in different women and not the screening result per se. Furthermore, recent published findings from the UKCTOCS data showed that screening does not necessarily provoke an unacceptable level of anxiety or psychological morbidity [77]. Taken together, these results support the position that surveillance and serial ultrasonography may not negatively impact perceptions of well-being, particularly if more women were made aware that some tumors may be low grade and slow growing.

6. Executive Summary of What We Already Know

There has been significant advancement in our understanding of ovarian cancer since the first randomized prospective ovarian cancer screen trials were initiated to detect cancers in early stages to reduce the mortality of this disease. We now know that ovarian cancer is a large heterogeneous group consisting of Type 1 (indolent and low grade tumor) and Type 2 (aggressive and high grade tumor) based on molecular, genetic make-up of the cancer and how they progress based on their precursors or genetic predisposition [16–32]. The evidence indicates that surgical treatment based on limited imaging or tumor marker data based on single or short-term exams has led to unnecessary surgery with potential for morbidity or mortality [34]. Ultrasounds in ovarian cancer screening have detected both Type 1 and Type 2 cancers even at early stages [5,12,35–38]. Because benign and malignant ovarian neoplasms share overlapping ultrasound morphologies, accounting for a high ratio of benign to malignant surgical findings and because ovarian cancer prevalence is low while the prevalence of ovarian abnormalities is high, active ultrasonographic surveillance of ovarian abnormalities based on the morphologic index provides the best means for detecting Type 2 ovarian cancers. Theoretical modeling on how Type 2 cancers behave has shown that it may be possible to detect low volume high grade cancer with better outcomes utilizing close follow-up with ultrasounds [46,47]. Ovarian cancer screening with ultrasound has detected a stage shift that finds malignancies at an earlier stage and serial ultrasound has increased the positive predictive value of this approach while decreasing false positive cases [5,36–38]. Medical-legal risk may enter the consideration when an indeterminate mass is not followed, often leading to surgery that proves unnecessary. Unnecessary surgery on false positive cases can have serious immediate complication rates ranging from 2–15% [12,34] but, if serial ultrasound indicates that the abnormality is resolving, then the need for surgery could be circumvented. Based on a comprehensive review of the literature, it can be concluded that:

(1) there are benefits in ultrasound monitoring of persisting indeterminate masses;
(2) resolution of sonographic abnormality defines benign status;
(3) stability over time may not equate with benign status particularly for Type 1 tumors;
(4) for certain types of tumors benign lesions are precursors of malignant lesions;
(5) repeated ultrasound monitoring does not negatively impact psychosocial well-being.

7. Conclusions

In conclusion, ultrasounds are inexpensive, associated with low morbidity, widely available, have high sensitivity in detecting abnormalities and are free of risk in image acquisition. Decisions for following ovarian masses detected by ultrasound in day-to-day practice differ from decisions for annual ovarian cancer screening in asymptomatic women with normal risk. The goal of ovarian cancer screening is to detect early stage ovarian cancer with improved mortality benefit. The role of ultrasounds in adnexal mass management should be to increase positive predictive value of detecting ovarian cancer to minimize unnecessary surgeries and to avoid failures to detect ovarian cancers. Findings from ovarian cancer screening trials and advances in our understanding of ovarian cancer pathogenesis can guide the management of adnexal masses found in clinical practice, especially since screening studies have observed that women with ovarian masses found by ultrasounds have a higher risk for ovarian cancer than those women who do not have an ovarian mass. Serial ultrasound surveillance using a morphologic index allows quantitative surveillance and the ability to distinguish benign masses based upon stable index scores (absence of growth, stable morphology) or decreasing index scores (resolution), while increasing index scores are strongly linked to malignancy. Concomitant use of serial CA-125 as in the ROCA model should also increase the positive predictive value of detecting malignancy. All improvements should promote a close working relationship between diagnostic radiology and clinicians using standardized structured reporting models as advocated by the American College of Radiology as seen in the Breast Imaging Reporting Data System (BI-RADS) or the Liver Imaging Reporting Data System (LI-RADS) to reduce ambiguous terminology, decrease variability in interpretation and improve communication.

Author Contributions: Eleanor L. Ormsby Edward J. Pavlik and John P. McGahan contributed equally to the writing, review and editing of this manuscript.

Conflicts of Interest: The authors declare no conflict of interest.

References

1. Siegel, R.L.; Miller, K.D.; Jemal, A. Cancer Statistics, 2015. *CA Cancer J. Clin.* **2015**, *65*, 5–29. [CrossRef] [PubMed]
2. U.S. Cancer Statistics Working Group. United States Cancer Statistics: 1999–2013 Incidence and Mortality Web-based Report. U.S. Department of Health and Human Services, Centers for Disease Control and Prevention and National Cancer Institute: Atlanta, 2016. Available online: www.cdc.gov/uscs (accessed on 25 April 2017).
3. American Cancer Society Surveillance Research 2015. Available online: http://www.cancer.org/acs/groups/content/@editorial/documents/document/acspc-044512.pdf (accessed on 25 April 2017).
4. Jemal, A.; Siegel, R.; Ward, E.; Murray, T.; Xu, J.; Thun, M.J. Cancer Statistics, 2007. *CA Cancer J. Clin.* **2007**, *57*, 43–66. [CrossRef] [PubMed]
5. Van Nagell, J.R., Jr.; Miller, R.W.; DeSimone, C.P.; Ueland, F.R.; Podzielinski, I.; Goodrich, S.T.; Elder, J.W.; Huang, B.; Kryscio, R.J.; Pavlik, E.J. Long-term survival of women with epithelial ovarian cancer detected by ultrasonographic screening. *Obstet. Gynecol.* **2011**, *118*, 1212–1221. [CrossRef]
6. Salani, R.; Bristow, R.E. Surgical management of epithelial ovarian cancer. *Clin. Obstet. Gynecol.* **2013**, *55*, 75–95. [CrossRef] [PubMed]
7. U.S. Preventive Services Task Force. Final Recommendation Statement Ovarian Cancer: Screening. September 2012. Available online: http://www.uspreventiveservicestaskforce.org/Page/Document/RecommendationStatementFinal/ovarian-cancer-screening (accessed on 29 December 2016).
8. Hartge, P.; Hayes, R.; Reding, D.; Sherman, M.E.; Prorok, P.; Schiffman, M.; Buys, S. Complex ovarian cysts in postmenopausal women are not associated with ovarian cancer risk factors: Preliminary data from the prostate, lung, colon, and ovarian cancer screening trial. *Am. J. Obstet. Gynecol.* **2000**, *183*, 1232–1237. [CrossRef] [PubMed]
9. Bailey, C.L.; Ueland, F.R.; Land, G.L.; DePriest, P.D.; Gallion, H.H.; Kryscio, R.J.; van Nagell, J.R., Jr. The malignant potential of small cystic ovarian tumors in women over 50 years of age. *Gynecol. Oncol.* **1998**, *69*, 3–7. [CrossRef] [PubMed]

10. Modesitt, S.C.; Pavlik, E.J.; Ueland, F.R.; DePriest, P.D.; Kryscio, R.J.; Nagell, J.R., Jr. Risk of malignancy in unilocular ovarian cystic tumors less than 10 centimeters in diameter. *Obstet. Gynecol.* **2003**, *102*, 594–599. [CrossRef]

11. Saunders, B.A.; Podzielinski, I.; Ware, R.A.; Goodrich, S.; Desimone, C.P.; Ueland, F.R.; Seamon, L.; Ubellacker, J.; Pavlik, E.J.; Kryscio, R.J.; et al. Risk of malignancy in sonographically confirmed septated cystic ovarian tumors. *Gynecol. Oncol.* **2010**, *118*, 278–282. [CrossRef] [PubMed]

12. Sharma, A.; Apostolidou, S.; Burnell, M.; Campbell, S.; Habib, M.; Gentry-Maharaj, A.; Amso, N.; Seif, M.W.; Fletcher, G.; Singh, N.; et al. Risk of epithelial ovarian cancer in asymptomatic women with ultrasound-detected ovarian masses: A prospective cohort study within the UK collaborative trial of ovarian cancer screening (UKCTOCS). *Ultrasound Obstet. Gynecol.* **2012**, *40*, 338–344. [CrossRef]

13. Ormsby, E.L.; Pavlik, E.J.; Van Nagell, J.R. Ultrasound follow up of an adnexal mass has the potential to save lives. *Am. J. Obstet. Gynecol.* **2015**, *213*, 657–661. [CrossRef] [PubMed]

14. Levine, D.; Brown, D.L.; Andreotti, R.F.; Benacerraf, B.; Benson, C.B.; Brewster, W.R.; Coleman, B.; DePriest, P.; Doubilet, P.M.; Goldstein, S.R.; et al. Society of Radiologists in Ultrasound. Management of asymptomatic ovarian and other adnexal cysts imaged at US Society of Radiologists in Ultrasound Consensus Conference Statement. *Radiology* **2010**, *26*, 121–131.

15. Glanc, P.; Benacerraf, B.; Bourne, T.; Brown, D.; Coleman, B.; Crum, C.; Dodge, J.; Levine, D.; Pavlik, E.; Timmerman, D.; et al. First International Consensus Report on Adnexal Masses: Management Recommendations. *J. Ultrasound Med.* **2017**. [CrossRef] [PubMed]

16. Kurman, R.J.; Shih, I. The origin and pathogenesis of epithelial ovarian cancer: A proposed unifying theory. *Am. J. Surg. Pathol.* **2010**, *34*, 433–443. [CrossRef] [PubMed]

17. Koshiyama, M.; Matsumura, N.; Konishi, I. Recent concepts of ovarian carcinogenesis: Type I and type II. *Biomed. Res. Int.* **2014**. [CrossRef] [PubMed]

18. Lim, D.; Olivia, D.E. Precursors and pathogenesis of ovarian carcinoma. *Pathology* **2013**, *45*, 229–242. [CrossRef] [PubMed]

19. Vang, R.; Shih, I.; Kurman, R.J. Ovarian low-grade and high-grade serous carcinoma: Pathogenesis, clinicopathologic and molecular biologic features, and diagnostic problems. *Adv. Anat. Pathol.* **2009**, *16*, 267–282. [CrossRef] [PubMed]

20. Cho, K.R.; Shih, I. Ovarian cancer. *Ann. Rev. Pathol.* **2009**, *4*, 287–313. [CrossRef] [PubMed]

21. Senturk, E.; Cohen, S.; Dottino, P.R.; Senturk, E.; Cohen, S.; Dottino, P.R.; Martignetti, J.A. A critical re-appraisal of *BRCA₁* methylation studies in ovarian cancer. *Gynecol. Oncol.* **2010**, *119*, 376–383. [CrossRef] [PubMed]

22. Alvarado-Cabrero, I.; Navani, S.S.; Young, R.H.; Scully, R.E. Tumors of the Fimbriated End of the Fallopian Tube: A Clinicopathologic Analysis of 20 Cases, Including Nine Carcinomas. *Int. J. Gynecol. Pathol.* **1997**, *16*, 189–196. [CrossRef] [PubMed]

23. Colgan, T.J.; Murphy, J.; Cole, D.E.; Narod, S.; Rosen, B. Occult carcinoma in prophylactic oophorectomy specimens: Prevalence and association with *BRCA* germline mutation status. *Am. J. Surg. Pathol.* **2001**, *25*, 1283–1289. [CrossRef] [PubMed]

24. Cass, I.; Holschneider, C.; Datta, N.; Barbuto, D.; Walts, A.E.; Karlan, B.Y. *BRCA*-mutation-associated fallopian tube carcinoma: A distinct clinical phenotype? *Obstet. Gynecol.* **2005**, *106*, 1327–1334. [CrossRef] [PubMed]

25. Medeiros, F.; Muto, M.G.; Lee, Y.; Elvin, J.A.; Callahan, M.J.; Feltmate, C.; Garber, J.E.; Cramer, D.W.; Crum, C.P. The tubal fimbria is a preferred site for early adenocarcinoma in women with familial ovarian cancer syndrome. *Am. J. Surg. Pathol.* **2006**, *30*, 230–236. [CrossRef] [PubMed]

26. Kindelberger, D.W.; Lee, Y.; Miron, A.; Hirsch, M.S.; Feltmate, C.; Medeiros, F.; Callahan, M.J.; Garner, E.O.; Gordon, R.W.; Birch, C.; et al. Intraepithelial Carcinoma of the Fimbriae and Pelvic Serous Carcinoma: Evidence for a Causal Relationship. *Am. J. Surg. Pathol.* **2007**, *31*, 161–169. [CrossRef] [PubMed]

27. Crum, C.R.; Drapkin, R.; Miron, A.; Ince, T.A.; Muto, M.; Kindelberger, D.W.; Lee, Y. The distal fallopian tube: A new model for pelvic serous carcinogenesis. *Curr. Opin. Obstet. Gynecol.* **2007**, *19*, 3–9. [CrossRef] [PubMed]

28. Guth, U.; Huang, D.J.; Bauer, G.; Stieger, M.; Wight, E.; Singer, G. Metastatic patterns at autopsy in patients with ovarian carcinoma. *Cancer* **2007**, *110*, 1272–1280. [CrossRef] [PubMed]

29. Landen, C.N.; Birrer, M.J.; Sood, A.K. Early Events in the Pathogenesis of Epithelial Ovarian Cancer. *J. Clin. Oncol.* **2008**, *26*, 995–1005. [CrossRef] [PubMed]

30. Lengyel, E. Ovarian Cancer Development and Metastasis. *Am. J. Pathol.* **2010**, *177*, 1053–1064. [CrossRef] [PubMed]

31. Crum, C.P.; Mckeon, F.D.; Xian, X. The oviduct and ovarian cancer: Causality, clinical implications, and "targeted prevention". *Clin. Obstet. Gynecol.* **2012**, *55*, 24–35. [CrossRef] [PubMed]

32. Malpica, A.; Deavers, M.T.; Lu, K.; Bodurka, D.C.; Atkinson, E.N.; Gershenson, D.M.; Silva, E.G. Grading ovarian serous carcinoma using a two-tier system. *Am. J. Surg. Pathol.* **2004**, *28*, 496–504. [CrossRef] [PubMed]

33. Kobayashi, H.; Yamada, Y.; Sado, T.; Sakata, M.; Yoshida, S.; Kawaguchi, R.; Kanayama, S.; Shigetomi, H.; Haruta, S.; Tsuji, Y.; et al. A randomized study of screening for ovarian cancer: A multicenter study in Japan. *Int. J. Gynecol. Cancer* **2008**, *18*, 414–420. [CrossRef] [PubMed]

34. Buys, S.S.; Partridge, E.; Black, A.; Johnson, C.C.; Lamerato, L.; Isaacs, C.; Reding, D.J.; Greenlee, R.T.; Yokochi, L.A.; Kessel, B.; et al. Effect of screening on ovarian cancer mortality: The Prostate, Lung, Colorectal and Ovarian (PLCO) Cancer Screening Randomized Controlled Trial. *JAMA* **2011**, *305*, 2295–2303. [CrossRef] [PubMed]

35. Jacobs, I.J.; Menon, U.; Ryan, A.; Gentry-Maharaj, A.; Burnell, M.; Kalsi, J.K. Ovarian cancer screening and mortality in the UK Collaborative Trial of Ovarian Cancer Screening (UKCTOCS): A randomised controlled trial. *Lancet* **2016**, *387*, 945–956. [CrossRef]

36. Pavlik, E.J.; Ueland, F.R.; Miller, R.W.; Ubellacker, J.M.; Desimone, C.P.; Elder, J.; Hoff, J.; Baldwin, L.; Kryscio, R.J.; van Nagell, J.R., Jr. Frequency and disposition of ovarian abnormalities followed with serial transvaginal ultrasonography. *Obstet. Gynecol.* **2013**, *122*, 210–217. [CrossRef] [PubMed]

37. Van Nagell, J.R., Jr.; Miller, R.W. Evaluation and Management of Ultrasonographically Detected Ovarian Tumors in Asymptomatic Women. *Obstet. Gynecol.* **2016**, *127*, 848–858. [CrossRef] [PubMed]

38. Van Nagell, J.R., Jr.; Hoff, J.T. Transvaginal ultrasonography in ovarian cancer screening: Current perspectives. *Int. J. Womens Health.* **2014**, *6*, 25–33. [CrossRef] [PubMed]

39. Elder, J.W.; Pavlik, E.J.; Long, A.; Miller, R.W.; Desimone, C.P.; Hoff, J.T.; Ueland, W.R.; Kryscio, R.J.; Nagell, J.R., Jr.; Ueland, F.R. Serial ultrasonographic evaluation of ovarian abnormalities with a morphology index. *Gynecol. Oncol.* **2014**, *135*, 8–12. [CrossRef] [PubMed]

40. Kaijser, J.; van Gorp, T.; van hoorde, k.; van Holsbeke, C.; Sayasneh, A.; Vergote, I.; Bourne, T.; Timmerman, D.; van Calster, B. A comparison between an ultrasound based prediction model (LR2) and the risk of ovarian malignancy algorithm (ROMA) to assess the risk of malignancy in women with an adnexal mass. *Gynecol. Oncol.* **2013**, *129*, 377–383. [CrossRef] [PubMed]

41. Urban, N.; Thorpe, J.D.; Bergan, L.A.; Forrest, R.M.; Kampani, A.V.; Scholler, N.; O'Briant, K.C.; Anderson, G.L.; Cramer, D.W.; Berg, C.D.; et al. Potential role of HE4 in multimodal screening for epithelial ovarian cancer. *J. Natl. Cancer Inst.* **2011**, *103*, 1630–1634. [CrossRef] [PubMed]

42. Moore, R.G.; MacLaughlan, S.; Bast, R.C. Current state of biomarker development for clinical application in epithelial ovarian cancer. *Gynecol. Oncol.* **2010**, *116*, 240–245. [CrossRef] [PubMed]

43. Skates, S.J.; Mai, P.; Horick, N.K.; Piedmonte, M.; Drescher, C.W.; Isaacs, C.; Armstrong, D.K.; Buys, S.S.; Rodriguez, G.C.; Horowitz, I.R.; et al. Large Prospective Study of Ovarian Cancer Screening in High risk Women: CA-125 Cut-point Defined by Menopausal Status. *Cancer Prev. Res. (Phila)* **2011**, *4*, 1401–1408. [CrossRef] [PubMed]

44. Menon, U.; Gentry-Maharaj, A.; Hallett, R.; Ryan, A.; Burnell, M.; Sharma, A.; Lewis, S.; Davies, S.; Philpott, S.; Lopes, A.; et al. Sensitivity and specificity of multimodal and ultrasound screening for ovarian cancer, and stage distribution of detected cancers: Results of the prevalence screen of the UK Collaborative Trial of Ovarian Cancer Screening (UKCTOCS). *Lancet Oncol.* **2009**, *10*, 327–340. [CrossRef]

45. Havrilesky, L.; Sanders, G.; Kulasingam, S.; Chino, J.; Berchuck, A.; Marks, J.; Evan, R.; Myers, E. Development of an ovarian cancer screening decision model that incorporates disease heterogeneity. *Cancer* **2010**, *117*, 545–553. [CrossRef] [PubMed]

46. Brown, P.O.; Palmer, C. The Preclinical Natural History of Serous Ovarian Cancer: Defining the Target for Early Detection. *PLoS Med.* **2009**, *6*. [CrossRef] [PubMed]

47. Hori, S.S.; Gambhir, S.S. Mathematical Model Identifies Blood Biomarker–Based Early Cancer Detection Strategies and Limitations. *Sci. Transl. Med.* **2011**, *3*, 109ra116.

48. Suh-Burgmann, E.; Hung, Y.Y.; Kinney, W. Outcomes from ultrasound follow-up of small complex adnexal masses in women over 50. *Am. J. Obstet. Gynecol.* **2014**, *211*, 623.e1–623.e7. [CrossRef] [PubMed]
49. Yazbek, J.; Raju, K.S.; Ben-Nagi, J.; Holland, T.; Hillaby, K.; Jurkovic, D. Accuracy of ultrasound subjective "pattern recognition" for the diagnosis of borderline ovarian tumors. *Ultrasound Obstet. Gynecol.* **2007**, *29*, 489–495. [CrossRef] [PubMed]
50. Valentin, L.; Ameye, L.; Franchi, D.; Guerriero, S.; Jurkovic, D.; Savell, L.; Fischerova, D.; Lissoni, A.; van Holsbeke, C.; Fruscio, R.; et al. Risk of malignancy in unilocular cysts: A study of 1148 adnexal masses classified as unilocular cysts at transvaginal ultrasound and review of the literature. *Ultrasound Obstet. Gynecol.* **2013**, *41*, 80–89. [CrossRef] [PubMed]
51. Yancik, R.; Ries, L.G.; Yates, J.W. Ovarian cancer in the elderly: An analysis of surveillance. *Am. J. Obstet. Gynecol.* **1986**, *154*, 639–647. [CrossRef]
52. Pavlik, E.J.; van Nagell, J.R. Early Detection of Ovarian Tumors Using Ultrasound. *Womens Health* **2013**, *9*, 39–55. [CrossRef] [PubMed]
53. Gilbert, L.; Basso, O.; Sampalis, J.; Karp, I.; Martins, C.; Feng, J.; Piedimonte, S.; Quintal, L.; Ramanakumar, A.V.; Takefman, J.; et al. Assessment of symptomatic women for early diagnosis of ovarian cancer: Results from the prospective DOvE pilot project. *Lancet Oncol.* **2012**, 285–291. [CrossRef]
54. Rossing, M.A.; Wicklund, K.G.; Cushing-Haugen, K.L.; Weiss, N.S. Predictive value of symptoms for early detection of ovarian cancer. *J. Natl. Cancer Inst.* **2010**, *102*, 222–229. [CrossRef] [PubMed]
55. Cooper, A.L.; Nelson, D.F.; Doran, S.; Ueland, F.R.; DeSimone, C.P.; DePriest, P.D.; McDonald, J.M.; Saunders, B.A.; Ware, R.A.; Pavlik, E.J.; et al. Long-Term Survival and Cost of Treatment in Patients with Stage IIIC Epithelial Ovarian Cancer. *Curr. Women's Health Rev.* **2009**, *5*, 44–50.
56. McColl, S.; Hicks, J.; Craig, L.; Shortreed, J. *Environmental Health Risk Management: A Primer for Canadians*; Graphic Services University of Waterloo: Waterloo, ON, Canada, 2000.
57. Zannoni, L.; Savelli, L.; Jokubkiene, L.; Di Legge, A.; Condous, G.; Testa, A.C.; Sladkevicius, P.; Valentin, L. Intra-and interobserver agreement with regard to describing adnexal masses using International Ovarian Tumor Analysis terminology: Reproducibility study involving seven observers. *Ultrasound Obstet. Gynecol.* **2014**, *44*, 100–108. [CrossRef] [PubMed]
58. Ueland, F.R.; DePriest, P.D.; Pavlik, E.J.; Kryscio, R.J.; Nagell, J.R., Jr. Preoperative differentiation of malignant from benign ovarian tumors: The efficacy of morphology indexing and Doppler flow sonography. *Gynecol. Oncol.* **2003**, *91*, 46–50. [CrossRef]
59. Testa, A.C.; Timmerman, D.; van Hosbeke, C.; Zannoni, G.F.; Fransis, S.; Moerman, P.; Vellone, V.; Mascilini, F.; Licameli, A.; Ludovisi, M.; et al. Ovarian cancer arising in endometrioid cysts: Ultrasound findings. *Ultrasound Obstet. Gynecol.* **2011**, *38*, 99–106. [CrossRef] [PubMed]
60. Fukunaga, M.; Nomura, K.; Ishikawa, E.; Ushigome, S. Ovarian atypical endometriosis: Its close association with malignant epithelial tumours. *Histopathology* **1997**, *30*, 249–255. [CrossRef] [PubMed]
61. Heaps, J.M.; Nieberg, R.K.; Berek, J.S. Malignant neoplasms arising in endometriosis. *Obstet. Gynecol.* **1990**, *75*, 1023–1028. [CrossRef]
62. Moll, U.M.; Chumas, J.C.; Chalas, E.; Mann, W.J. Ovarian carcinoma arising in atypical endometriosis. *Obstet. Gynecol.* **1990**, *75*, 537–539. [PubMed]
63. Sainz de la Cuesta, R.; Eichhorn, J.H.; Rice, L.W.; Fuller, A.F., Jr.; Nikrui, N.; Goff, B.A. Histologic transformation of benign endometriosis to early epithelial ovarian cancer. *Gynecol. Oncol.* **1996**, *60*, 238–244. [CrossRef] [PubMed]
64. Stern, R.C.; Dash, R.; Bentley, R.C.; Snyder, M.J.; Haney, A.F.; Robboy, S.J. Malignancy in endometriosis: Frequency and comparison of ovarian and extraovarian types. *Int. J. Gynecol. Pathol.* **2001**, *20*, 133–139. [PubMed]
65. Ogawa, S.; Kaku, T.; Amada, S.; Kobayashi, H.; Hirakawa, T.; Ariyoshi, K.; Kamura, T.; Nakano, H. Ovarian endometriosis associated with ovarian carcinoma: A clinicopathological and immunohistochemical study. *Gynecol. Oncol.* **2000**, *77*, 298–304. [CrossRef] [PubMed]
66. Mostoufizadeh, M.; Scully, R.E. Malignant tumors arising in endometriosis. *Clin. Obstet. Gynecol.* **1980**, *23*, 951–963. [CrossRef] [PubMed]
67. Russell, P. The pathological assessment of ovarian neoplasms. I: Introduction to the common "epithelial" tumours and analysis of benign "epithelial" tumours. *Pathology* **1979**, *11*, 5–26. [CrossRef] [PubMed]

68. Bell, D.A.; Scully, R.E. Atypical and borderline endometrioid adenofibromas of the ovary: A report of 27 cases. *Am. J. Surg. Pathol.* **1985**, *9*, 205–214. [CrossRef] [PubMed]
69. Snyder, R.R.; Norris, H.J.; Tavassoli, F. Endometrioid proliferative and low malignant potential tumors of the ovary: A clinicopathologic study of 46 cases. *Am. J. Surg. Pathol.* **1988**, *12*, 661–671. [CrossRef] [PubMed]
70. Pavlik, E.J.; van Nagell, J.R., Jr. Ovarian cancer screening—What women want. *Int. J. Gynecol. Cancer* **2012**, *22*, S21–S23. [CrossRef] [PubMed]
71. Salsman, J.M.; Pavlik, E.; Boerner, L.M.; Andrykowski, M.A. Clinical, demographic, and psychological characteristics of new, asymptomatic partipants in a transvaginal ultrasound screening program for ovarian cancer. *Prev. Med.* **2004**, *39*, 315–322. [CrossRef] [PubMed]
72. Lykins, E.L.; Pavlik, E.; Andrykowski, M.A. Validity of self-reports of return for routine repeat screening in an ovarian screening program. *Cancer Epidemiol. Biomark. Prev.* **2007**, *16*, 490–493. [CrossRef] [PubMed]
73. Gaugler, J.E.; Pavlik, E.; Salsman, J.M.; Andrykowski, M.A. Psychological and behavioral impact of receipt of a "normal" ovarian cancer screening test. *Prev. Med.* **2006**, *42*, 463–470. [CrossRef] [PubMed]
74. Andrykowski, M.A.; Boerner, L.M.; Salsman, J.M.; Pavlik, E. Psychological response to test results in an ovarian cancer screening program: A prospective, longitudinal study. *Health Psychol.* **2004**, *23*, 622–666. [CrossRef] [PubMed]
75. Ryan, P.Y.; Graves, K.D.; Pavlik, E.J.; Andrykowski, M.A. Abnormal ovarian cancer screening test result: Women's informational, psychological and practical needs. *J. Psychosoc. Oncol.* **2007**, *25*, 1–18. [CrossRef] [PubMed]
76. Andrykowski, M.A.; Pavlik, E. Response to an abnormal ovarian cancer-screening test result: Test of the social cognitive processing and cognitive social health information processing models. *Psychol. Health* **2011**, *26*, 383–397. [CrossRef] [PubMed]
77. Barrett, J.; Jenkins, V.; Farewell, V. BJOG: Psychological morbidity associated with ovarian cancer screening: Results from more than 23,000 women in the randomised trial of ovarian cancer screening (UKCTOCS). *BJOG* **2014**, *121*, 1071–1079. [CrossRef] [PubMed]

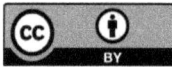

MDPI

Article

Validation of the Performance of International Ovarian Tumor Analysis (IOTA) Methods in the Diagnosis of Early Stage Ovarian Cancer in a Non-Screening Population

Wouter Froyman [1,2], Laure Wynants [1], Chiara Landolfo [1,2], Tom Bourne [1,2,3], Lil Valentin [4], Antonia Testa [5], Povilas Sladkevicius [4], Dorella Franchi [6], Daniela Fischerova [7], Luca Savelli [8], Ben Van Calster [1] and Dirk Timmerman [1,2,*]

[1] Department of Development and Regeneration, KU Leuven, Leuven post code3000, Belgium; wouter.froyman@uzleuven.be (W.F.); laure.wynants@kuleuven.be (L.W.); chiara.landolfo@kuleuven.be (C.L.); t.bourne@imperial.ac.uk (T.B.); ben.vancalster@kuleuven.be (B.V.C.)

[2] Department of Obstetrics and Gynecology, University Hospitals Leuven, Leuven 3000, Belgium

[3] Queen Charlotte's and Chelsea Hospital, Imperial College, London W12 0HS, UK

[4] Department of Obstetrics and Gynecology, Skåne University Hospital Malmö, Lund University, Malmö 20502, Sweden; lil.valentin@med.lu.se (L.V.); povilas.sladkevicius@med.lu.se (P.S.)

[5] Department of Oncology, Catholic University of the Sacred Heart, Rome 00168, Italy; atesta@rm.unicatt.it

[6] Preventive Gynecology Unit, Division of Gynecology, European Institute of Oncology, Milan 20141, Italy; dorella.franchi@ieo.it

[7] Gynecological Oncology Center, Department of Obstetrics and Gynecology, Charles University, Prague 12108, Czech Republic; Daniela.Fischerova@seznam.cz

[8] Department of Obstetrics and Gynecology, S. Orsola-Malpighi Hospital, University of Bologna, Bologna 40138, Italy; luca.savelli@aosp.bo.it

* Correspondence: dirk.timmerman@uzleuven.be; Tel.: +32-16-3-44201 or +32-16-3-44216

Academic Editor: Edward J. Pavlik
Received: 28 March 2017; Accepted: 26 May 2017; Published: 2 June 2017

Abstract: Background: The aim of this study was to assess and compare the performance of different ultrasound-based International Ovarian Tumor Analysis (IOTA) strategies and subjective assessment for the diagnosis of early stage ovarian malignancy. Methods: This is a secondary analysis of a prospective multicenter cross-sectional diagnostic accuracy study that included 1653 patients recruited at 18 centers from 2009 to 2012. All patients underwent standardized transvaginal ultrasonography by experienced ultrasound investigators. We assessed test performance of the IOTA Simple Rules (SRs), Simple Rules Risk (SRR), the Assessment of Different NEoplasias in the adneXa (ADNEX) model and subjective assessment to discriminate between stage I-II ovarian cancer and benign disease. Reference standard was histology after surgery. Results: 230 (13.9%) patients proved to have stage I–II primary invasive ovarian malignancy, and 1423 (86.1%) had benign disease. Sensitivity and specificity with respect to malignancy (95% confidence intervals) of the original SRs (classifying all inconclusive cases as malignant) were 94.3% (90.6% to 96.7%) and 73.4% (71.0% to 75.6%). Subjective assessment had a sensitivity and specificity of 90.0% (85.4% to 93.2%) and 86.7% (84.9% to 88.4%), respectively. The areas under the receiver operator characteristic curves of SRR and ADNEX were 0.917 (0.902 to 0.933) and 0.905 (0.920 to 0.934), respectively. At a 1% risk cut-off, sensitivity and specificity for SRR were 100% (98.4% to 100%) and 38.0% (35.5% to 40.6%), and for ADNEX were 100% (98.4% to 100%) and 19.4% (17.4% to 21.5%). At a 30% risk cut-off, sensitivity and specificity for SRR were 88.3% (83.5% to 91.8%) and 81.1% (79% to 83%), and for ADNEX were 84.5% (80.5% to 89.6%) and 84.5% (82.6% to 86.3%). Conclusion: This study shows that all three IOTA strategies have good ability to discriminate between stage I-II ovarian malignancy and benign disease.

Keywords: ovary; ovarian neoplasms; early detection of cancer; diagnostic imaging; ultrasonography; risk assessment; logistic models

---

1. Introduction

Ovarian tumors are common in women of all ages [1–3]. It has been estimated that in the female population, the lifetime risk of undergoing surgery for a suspected ovarian neoplasm is 5–10% [4]. However, the incidence of ovarian cancer is low. In Europe, there were 65,538 new cases during 2012, with an age-adjusted incidence rate of 13.1 per 100,000 women. Still, ovarian cancer is an important health problem in gynecology, as it is the most lethal gynecological malignancy, with 42,700 deaths occurring in 2012 in Europe (mortality rate 7.6 per 100,000) [5]. This accounts for 5% of all cancer deaths in women, which makes ovarian cancer the sixth most lethal cancer in females in Europe [6].

In recent decades, despite advances in cytoreductive radical surgery and cytotoxic chemotherapy, we have seen only a marginal improvement in the overall survival of patients with ovarian cancer [7].

Almost 60% of patients are diagnosed with advanced disease with regional or distant spread and an unfavorable long-term prognosis. Five-year relative survival is 46% for all International Federation of Gynecology and Obstetrics (FIGO) stages [8], but ranges from 90% at Stage I to 4% for Stage IV disease [6,8]. Therefore, attention for the development of strategies to detect ovarian malignancy at an early stage using imaging and/or biomarkers is increasing, in order to improve patient survival. This idea is reflected in the conduction of several large ovarian cancer screening trials [9–11], but also plays an important role in clinical management of the non-screening population.

Early detection of cancer means that treatment is not delayed and that appropriate staging can be carried out in specialized surgical centers, which is known to improve survival [12–15].

The best ultrasound method for discrimination between benign and malignant adnexal masses is the subjective assessment of ultrasound findings by an experienced ultrasound examiner [16–18]. However, as such expert knowledge is not available in each center, the International Ovarian Tumor Analysis (IOTA) study aims to develop diagnostic algorithms to assist clinicians in characterizing adnexal pathology, irrespective of their level of expertise. The IOTA group initially published a consensus paper in order to standardize terms, definitions, and measurements used to assess ovarian pathology [19]. By prospectively investigating patients presenting with an adnexal mass (i.e., non-screening population), this formed the basis for the development of different IOTA methods such as the Simple Rules (SRs), which are based on five ultrasound features suggestive for a benign lesion (B-features) and five features suggestive for a malignant lesion (M-features) [20]. The IOTA SRs have become very popular because they are easy to use, without the need for any calculation. They have been extensively validated and are incorporated in international guidelines [21,22]. Two systematic reviews and meta-analyses have concluded that the IOTA SRs are one of the best performing available diagnostic methods for differentiating between benign and malignant adnexal masses [18,23]. Shortcomings of the SRs are that there are inconclusive results in a proportion of cases (when B and M features apply or when no features apply) and the absence of an estimated risk of malignancy. Therefore, the ultrasound features used in the SRs have recently been used to calculate a risk of malignancy, leading to the Simple Rules Risk (SRR) model [24]. Another logistic regression model developed by the IOTA group is the Assessment of Different NEoplasias in the adneXa (ADNEX) model. As a multiclass prediction model, ADNEX not only calculates the likelihood of malignancy in adnexal masses, but also divides this into the likelihood that the mass is borderline malignant, stage I primary invasive ovarian cancer, stage II–IV primary invasive ovarian cancer, or a metastasis in the ovary from another primary tumor [25]. The performance of ADNEX is at least as good as the performance of previous IOTA methods, as confirmed by external validation studies [26–30]. The ADNEX model is available online and in mobile applications (www.iotagroup.org/adnexmodel/).

Given the good performance of IOTA strategies in discriminating between benign and malignant disease in patients presenting with an adnexal mass prior to surgery, we are often confronted with the question on how IOTA methods could potentially improve detection in ovarian cancer screening. For the purpose of this special issue of Diagnostics, we assessed and compared the test performance of various diagnostic IOTA methods and subjective assessment to identify early stage, i.e., FIGO stage I and II [8], primary invasive ovarian malignancy in a non-screening population.

2. Materials and Methods

2.1. Patients

This study was performed on data of IOTA phase 3 [31], a multicenter cross-sectional diagnostic accuracy study with prospective data collection. Patients were recruited in 18 centers in six countries (Sweden, Belgium, Italy, Poland, Spain, and Czech Republic) between October 2009 and May 2012. The participating centers were either oncology referral centers (i.e., tertiary centers with a specific gynecological oncology unit) or general hospitals and units with a special interest in gynecological ultrasound. Ethics approval for IOTA 3 was obtained by the ethics committee of the University Hospitals Leuven (B32220095331/S51375 approved 21 January 2009) as the main investigating center as well of the local ethics committees of all contributing centers.

Patients were eligible for IOTA 3 if they presented with at least one adnexal mass (ovarian, para-ovarian, or tubal), underwent standardized transvaginal ultrasonography by a principal investigator at one of the participating centers, and were then selected for surgical intervention by the managing clinician. All examiners were experienced in gynecologic ultrasound. Details on the ultrasound examination technique and the IOTA terms and definitions used to describe adnexal pathology have been published elsewhere [19]. More information on data collection can be found in the original IOTA 3 publication [31]. The pathologist was blinded to the predicted outcomes of the index tests being compared.

For the purpose this study, only patients having a histopathology diagnosis of a benign mass or FIGO stage I and II [8] invasive (epithelial or non-epithelial) ovarian malignancy were considered for analysis.

2.2. Diagnostic Models

Three diagnostic IOTA methods for the assessment of adnexal masses (the original SRs, SRR and ADNEX) were evaluated in terms of their ability to discriminate between benign disease and stage I–II primary ovarian malignancy. These methods were developed on data of earlier IOTA phases. Hence, this is a temporal validation study, including new centers. The original IOTA SRs result in a classification of ovarian masses as benign, malignant, or inconclusive. In this work, we classified inconclusive cases as malignant. The SRR yields a predicted probability of ovarian malignancy. The ADNEX model provides the predicted risks of four different subclasses of malignant adnexal tumors (borderline, stage I invasive, stage II-IV invasive or metastatic cancer). When using the ADNEX model, the probability of malignancy is computed as the sum of the predicted probabilities for all malignant subtypes (including borderline tumors). We validated the version of ADNEX that does not use serum cancer antigen 125 (CA125) measurements as a predictor, because CA125 results are not always available in women with benign or stage I–II tumors (results for serum CA125 measurements were missing for 45% of women in our database). ADNEX with and without CA125 has similar ability to predict malignancy [25]. Both SRR and ADNEX were initially developed on data from IOTA phases 1 and 2, validated on data from IOTA 3, and then refitted on all data [24,25]. In this study, we used the initial versions of SRR and ADNEX that were not refitted using IOTA 3 data. We also evaluated the performance of subjective assessment.

2.3. Statistical Methods

All strategies were evaluated in terms of their ability to discriminate between benign and malignant masses. The area under the receiver-operator characteristic curve (AUC) was computed for ADNEX and the SRR. We also calculated the sensitivity and specificity for ADNEX and the SRR at risk thresholds of 1%, 10%, 20%, and 30%, as well the sensitivity and specificity of the original SRs (classifying inconclusive results as malignant) and subjective assessment. Subgroup analyses were performed for pre- and postmenopausal women. R software (version 3.3.1.) was used for all calculations (R: A language and environment for statistical computing. R Foundation for Statistical Computing, Vienna, Austria, Available online: http/www.r-project.org/). The pROC package and binom packages were used to calculate Delong [32] and Wilson [33] confidence intervals for AUCs and sensitivity/specificity, respectively. The Transparent Reporting of a multivariable prediction model for Individual Prognosis or Diagnosis (TRIPOD) guidelines [34] were used for reporting in this study.

3. Results

In total, 2541 women with adnexal masses were enrolled in IOTA phase 3. We excluded 138 women from the final data set after the application of exclusion criteria [31].

Of the remaining 2403 patients, 1423 had a benign mass. Patients with borderline tumors, stage III–IV primary invasive malignancies, and metastatic cancer were excluded from the analysis. The resulting database for analysis consisted of 1653 women from 18 centers, 230 of which had stage I–II invasive ovarian malignancy. Patient and tumor characteristics are represented in Table 1. Of the women included, 34.6% were postmenopausal. Histology findings are listed in Table 2.

Table 1. Descriptive statistics of the sample.

Variable	Result	
	Benign Tumor	**Early Stage Malignancy (I and II)**
N	1423 (86.1%)	230 (13.9%)
Age (years)	44 (33 to 56)	55 (42 to 66)
Postmenopausal	447 (31.4%)	125 (54.3%)
CA125 (IU/L), if available [a]	21 (12 to 46)	55 (20 to 207)
Maximum tumor diameter (mm)	64 (47 to 90)	103 (68 to 143)
Presence of solid components	474 (33.3%)	214 (93.0%)
Maximum diameter of the solid component (if any, mm)	28 (13 to 54)	62 (37 to 93)
Locularity		
Unilocular	595 (41.8%)	2 (0.9%)
Unilocular-solid	141 (9.9%)	34 (14.8%)
Multilocular	354 (24.9%)	14 (6.1%)
Multilocular-solid	179 (12.6%)	93 (40.4%)
Solid	154 (10.8%)	87 (37.8%)
Number of locules (if any)	1 (1 to 3)	5 (1.5 to 6)
Acoustic shadows	265 (18.6%)	17 (7.4%)
Intratumoral blood flow		
No blood flow	574 (40.3%)	5 (2.2%)
Minimal blood flow	563 (39.6%)	54 (23.5%)
Moderate blood flow	239 (16.8%)	95 (41.3%)
Very strong blood flow	47 (3.3%)	76 (33.0%)
Irregular internal cyst wall	385 (27.1%)	151 (65.7%)
Presence of ascites	18 (1.3%)	33 (14.3%)
Presence of papillary structures	180 (12.6%)	54 (23.5%)
Number of papillary structures (if present)	1 (1 to 3)	3 (2 to 4)

[a] CA125: cancer antigen 125. There were 683 (48%) missing values for CA125 for benign tumors and 64 (28%) for early stage tumors.

Results are shown as medians (interquartile range) for continuous and ordinal variables, and as *N* (%) for categorical variables. Possible values for "Number of locules" are 1 = presence of one locule,

2 = presence of two locules, 3 = presence of three locules, 4 = presence of four locules, 5 = presence of five to ten locules, 6 = presence of more than ten locules. Possible values for "Number of papillary structures" are 1 = presence of one papillary structure, 2 = presence of two papillary structures, 3 = presence of three papillary structures, 4 = presence of more than three papillary structures.

Table 2. Overview of histologic outcomes (*N*, %).

Histology	N (%)
Endometrioma	344 (20.8%)
Teratoma	231 (14.0%)
Simple cyst + parasalpingeal cyst	106 (6.4%)
Functional cyst	40 (2.4%)
Hydrosalpinx + salpingitis	47 (2.8%)
Peritoneal pseudocyst	18 (1.1%)
Abscess	17 (1.0%)
Fibroma	130 (7.9%)
Serous cystadenoma	259 (15.7%)
Mucinous cystadenoma	183 (11.1%)
Rare benign	48 (2.9%)
Primary invasive (epithelial) cancer stage I	128 (7.7%)
Primary invasive (epithelial) cancer stage II	47 (2.8%)
Rare primary invasive malignancy stage I or II *	55 (3.3%)

* Includes germ cell tumors and sex cord-stromal tumors.

Regarding the identification of stage I–II primary ovarian malignancy as malignant disease, the original SRs (classifying inconclusive cases as malignant) had a sensitivity and specificity (95% confidence intervals) of 94.3% (90.6% to 96.7%) and 73.4% (71.0% to 75.6%). Subjective assessment had a sensitivity and specificity of 90.0% (85.4% to 93.2%) and 86.7% (84.9% to 88.4%), respectively. Considering the discrimination of benign and malignant disease in the study population of patients with benign masses and stage I–II primary ovarian malignancy the AUCs of the SRR and ADNEX model were 0.917 (0.902 to 0.933) and 0.920 (0.905 to 0.934), respectively. The sensitivity and specificity for these risk prediction models differ depending on the selected risk threshold to predict malignancy. Table 3 summarizes the sensitivity and specificity for the two models at different risk thresholds.

Table 3. Sensitivity and specificity for Assessment of Different NEoplasias in the adneXa (ADNEX) model and Simple Rules Risk (SRR) model at various risk thresholds (percent (95% confidence interval)).

Risk Threshold	Statistic	ADNEX	SRR
1%	Sensitivity	100.0% (98.4% to 100.0%)	100.0% (98.4% to 100.0%)
	Specificity	19.4% (17.4% to 21.5%)	38.0% (35.5% to 40.6%)
10%	Sensitivity	97.4% (94.4% to 98.8%)	97.0% (93.9% to 98.5%)
	Specificity	69.5% (67.1% to 71.8%)	65.1% (62.6% to 67.6%)
20%	Sensitivity	91.3% (87.0% to 94.3%)	94.3% (90.6% to 96.7%)
	Specificity	79.7% (77.5% to 81.7%)	74.3% (71.9% to 76.5%)
30%	Sensitivity	84.5% (80.5% to 89.6%)	88.3% (83.5% to 91.8%)
	Specificity	84.5% (82.6% to 86.3%)	81.1% (79.0% to 83.0%)

When stratifying for menopausal status, the original SRs (classifying inconclusive cases as malignant) had a sensitivity and specificity of 94.3% (88.1% to 97.4%) and 77.3% (74.5% to 79.8%) in premenopausal patients, and 94.4% (88.9% to 97.3%) and 64.9% (60.3% to 69.2%) in postmenopausal patients. Subjective assessment had a sensitivity and specificity of 87.6% (80.0% to 92.6%) and 89.0% (86.9% to 90.8%) in premenopausal patients, and 92.0% (85.9% to 95.6%) and 81.7% (77.8% to 85.0%) in postmenopausal patients.

In premenopausal women, the AUCs of the SRR and ADNEX model were 0.932 (0.913 to 0.950) and 0.932 (0.913 to 0.950), respectively. In postmenopausal women, the AUCs of the SRR and ADNEX model were 0.882 (0.853 to 0.912) and 0.885 (0.858 to 0.912), respectively.

Table 4 summarizes the sensitivity and specificity for the two models at different risk thresholds for pre- and postmenopausal women.

Table 4. Sensitivity and specificity by menopausal status for Assessment of Different NEoplasias in the adneXa (ADNEX) model and Simple Rules Risk (SRR) model at various risk thresholds (percent (95% confidence interval)).

Risk Threshold	Statistic	ADNEX		SRR	
		Premenopausal	Postmenopausal	Premenopausal	Postmenopausal
1%	Sens	100.0% (96.5% to 100.0%)	100.0% (97.0% to 100%)	100.0% (96.5% to 100.0%)	100% (97.0% to 100.0%)
	Spec	25.8% (23.2% to 28.7%)	5.4% (3.6% to 7.9%)	41.4% (38.3% to 44.5%)	30.6% (26.6% to 35.1%)
10%	Sens	94.3% (88.1% to 97.4%)	100% (97.0% to 100%)	98.1% (93.3% to 99.5%)	96.0% (91.0% to 98.3%)
	Spec	77.8% (75.1% to 80.3%)	51.5% (46.8% to 56.1%)	70.6% (67.7% to 73.4%)	53.2% (48.6% to 57.8%)
20%	Sens	86.7% (78.9% to 91.9%)	95.2% (89.9% to 97.8%)	94.3% (88.1% to 97.4%)	94.4% (88.9% to 97.3%)
	Spec	85.6% (83.2% to 87.6%)	66.9% (62.4% to 71.1%)	78.5% (75.8% to 80.9%)	65.1% (60.6% to 69.4%)
30%	Sens	78.1% (69.3% to 84.9%)	92.0% (85.9% to 95.6%)	84.8% (76.7% to 90.4%)	91.2% (84.9% to 95.0%)
	Spec	89.5% (87.5% to 81.3%)	73.6% (96.3% to 77.5%)	84.1% (81.7% to 86.3%)	74.5% (70.3% to 78.3%)

4. Discussion

This validation of IOTA ultrasound-based rules and risk prediction models showed good test performance to discriminate between benign disease and stage I–II ovarian malignancy before surgery.

The strength of this study is the use of a large international database in which information was prospectively collected using well-defined terms, definitions, and measurement methods [19]. The large sample size and the participation of different types of centers are likely to yield generalizable results.

A limitation of our study is that the diagnostic methods were validated exclusively on patients who underwent surgery. This does not reflect clinical practice, where some masses are managed expectantly, but it allowed us to use histological diagnosis as the gold standard. We are awaiting the results of IOTA phase 5, in which IOTA methods are validated on consecutively collected adnexal masses of all kinds, including those managed conservatively. A second limitation is that all ultrasound examiners in the study were very experienced. Our results might not necessarily be applicable to less experienced operators. However, published studies have shown that the IOTA SRs and ADNEX retain their performance in the hands of less experienced examiners [27,28,35–41]. This is likely to be true also for the SRR model, because the same ultrasound variables are used in the original SRs are used to calculate the risks of the SRR model. A third limitation of our study is that not all histopathology information necessary to classify the tumors into type I and type II epithelial malignancies had been collected. This is explained by the fact that patient recruitment for IOTA 3 started in 2009, before the dualistic model of ovarian carcinogenesis [42] was widely accepted.

The findings of our study show that the performance of IOTA methods for differentiating benign disease from stage I–II primary ovarian malignancy is not much lower than the performance

Diagnostics **2017**, *7*, 32

for the discrimination of benign from all malignant disease (all malignant subtypes grouped together) [24,25,31]. In the original publications including all IOTA 3 patients, validation AUCs (95% confidence intervals) regarding discrimination between benign and malignant disease for SRR and ADNEX (without CA125) were 0.917 (0.902–0.930) [24] and 0.932 (0.922–0.941) [25], respectively. Sensitivity and specificity for the original SRs on validation in the same population were 95.3% (93.1% to 96.9%) and 74.1% (67.7% to 79.7%), respectively [24,25,31].

Borderline malignant tumors were excluded from our analysis. These tumors are known to be more difficult to classify as benign or malignant [25,43,44]. On the other hand, borderline (i.e., non-invasive malignant) ovarian tumors rarely precede invasive epithelial ovarian carcinoma [45,46]. More clinically relevant is the correct identification of early stage primary invasive tumors, where prompt and adequate surgical staging is important for improving survival [47]. Detection of stage I-II ovarian cancer is particularly important for screening for ovarian cancer to be successful. The aim of screening for ovarian cancer is to decrease ovarian cancer mortality. For this to be possible, screening should result in a shift towards earlier stages at detection, i.e., the detection rate of stage I–II ovarian cancer should be high. However, a shift towards earlier detection of ovarian cancer has been shown in only two [9,11] of three randomized controlled trials [9–11] on ovarian cancer screening, and none of the two completed screening trials has shown conclusive evidence of decreased ovarian cancer mortality in the screened group [10,11]. In the two completed randomized trials on ovarian cancer screening [10,11], the ultrasound criteria to define an abnormal screening result were subjective or arbitrary. As a result, many patients with benign disease were scheduled for surgery, i.e., a large number of operations were performed to detect one cancer case. We speculate that the positive predictive value of an abnormal screen result could be improved if the IOTA methods were used to define an abnormal scan result. To the best of our knowledge, the discriminative or predictive performance of the IOTA methods has never been assessed in a screening population.

About 90% of invasive malignant ovarian tumors are epithelial [48]. The dualistic model proposed by Shih and Kurman highlights the heterogeneity of ovarian carcinoma and implies that ultrasound-based screening will not be effective in detecting all types of ovarian carcinoma. Type I tumors (low-grade serous, low-grade endometrioid, clear cell, and mucinous) are slow growing, attain a large size while still confined to the ovary, and are thus likely to be detected early by transvaginal ultrasound. Unfortunately, these lesions constitute only 25% of ovarian cancers and account for only approximately 10% of ovarian cancer deaths. On the other hand, type II tumors (high-grade serous and undifferentiated carcinomas, and malignant mixed mesodermal tumors (carcinosarcomas)) represent 75% of all ovarian carcinomas, are responsible for 90% of ovarian cancer deaths, and may originate outside the ovary. These tumors are almost never confined to the ovary at diagnosis, making their diagnosis at an early point in the disease course challenging [42,49]. To allow detection of this aggressive type of ovarian cancer, there is ongoing search for sensitive biomarkers expressed early in ovarian carcinogenesis. More recently, there is increasing interest in the use of genomic profiling as a potential candidate for the detection of ovarian malignancies [50,51]. Further research should explore whether IOTA methods may serve as a second stage test in a program of ovarian cancer screening to avoid unnecessary surgery without delaying a diagnosis of ovarian cancer.

5. Conclusions

This analysis shows that the IOTA methods have good ability to discriminate between stage I–II ovarian malignancy and benign adnexal lesions prior to surgery. The potential use of IOTA methods as a second stage test in ovarian cancer screening should be the subject of further investigation.

Acknowledgments: This study was supported by the Flemish government (Research Foundation–Flanders (FWO) project G049312N and G0B4716N, Flanders' Agency for Innovation by Science and Technology (IWT) project IWT-TBM 070706-IOTA3, and iMinds 2015) and Internal Funds KU Leuven (University of Leuven) (project C24/15/037). Dirk Timmerman is a senior clinical investigator of Fonds Wetenschappelijk Onderzoek (FWO). Tom Bourne is supported by the National Institute for Health Research (NIHR) Biomedical Research Centre based at Imperial College Healthcare National Health Service (NHS) Trust and Imperial College London.

The views expressed are those of the authors and not necessarily those of the NHS, NIHR or Department of Health, Lil Valentin is supported by the Swedish Medical Research Council (grants K2001-72X-11605-06A, K2002-72X-11605-07B, K2004-73X-11605-09A, and K2006-73X-11605-11-3), funds administered by Malmö University Hospital and Skåne University Hospital, Allmänna Sjukhusets i Malmö Stiftelse för bekämpande av cancer (the Malmö General Hospital Foundation for fighting against cancer), and two Swedish governmental grants (Avtal om läkarutbildning och forskning (ALF)-medel and Landstingsfinansierad Regional Forskning). Laure Wynants holds a postdoctoral mandate from Internal Funds KU Leuven. The sponsors had no role in study design; in the collection, analysis, and interpretation of data; in the writing of the report; and in the decision to submit the work for publication. The researchers performed this work independently of the funding sources.

Author Contributions: Wouter Froyman, Laure Wynants, Chiara Landolfo, Ben Van Calster and Dirk Timmerman conceived and designed the study, with additional support from Tom Bourne, Lil Valentin and Antonia Testa; Lil Valentin, Antonia Testa, Povilas Sladkevicius, Dorella Franchi, Daniela Fischerova, Luca Savelli and Dirk Timmerman enrolled patients and acquired data; Ben Van Calster and Dirk Timmerman were involved in data cleaning; Laure Wynants analyzed the data, with support from Ben Van Calster; Wouter Froyman, Laure Wynants, Chiara Landolfo, Tom Bourne, Lil Valentin, Antonia Testa, Ben Van Calster and Dirk Timmerman were involved in data interpretation; Wouter Froyman, Laure Wynants, Chiara Landolfo, Ben Van Calster and Dirk Timmerman wrote the first draft of the manuscript, which was then critically reviewed and revised by the other coauthors. All authors approved the final version of the manuscript for submission; Laure Wynants, Ben Van Calster and Dirk Timmerman had full access to all the data in the study and take responsibility for the integrity of the data and the accuracy of the data analysis.

Conflicts of Interest: The authors declare no conflict of interest.

References

1. Pavlik, E.J.; Ueland, F.R.; Miller, R.W.; Ubellacker, J.M.; DeSimone, C.P.; Elder, J.; Hoff, J.; Baldwin, L.; Kryscio, R.J.; van Nagell, J.R., Jr. Frequency and disposition of ovarian abnormalities followed with serial transvaginal ultrasonography. *Obstet. Gynecol.* **2013**, *122*, 210–217. [CrossRef] [PubMed]

2. Castillo, G.; Alcazar, J.L.; Jurado, M. Natural history of sonographically detected simple unilocular adnexal cysts in asymptomatic postmenopausal women. *Gynecol. Oncol.* **2004**, *92*, 965–969. [CrossRef] [PubMed]

3. Borgfeldt, C.; Andolf, E. Transvaginal sonographic ovarian findings in a random sample of women 25–40 years old. *Ultrasound Obstet. Gynecol.* **1999**, *13*, 345–350. [CrossRef] [PubMed]

4. Curtin, J.P. Management of the Adnexal Mass. *Gynecol. Oncol.* **1994**, *55*, S42–S46. [CrossRef] [PubMed]

5. Ferlay, J.; Steliarova-Foucher, E.; Lortet-Tieulent, J.; Rosso, S.; Coebergh, J.W.; Comber, H.; Forman, D.; Bray, F. Cancer incidence and mortality patterns in Europe: Estimates for 40 countries in 2012. *Eur. J. Cancer* **2013**, *49*, 1374–1403. [CrossRef] [PubMed]

6. Cancer Research UK. Available online: www.cancerresearchuk.org (accessed on 20 November 2016).

7. Vaughan, S.; Coward, J.I.; Bast, R.C., Jr.; Berchuck, A.; Berek, J.S.; Brenton, J.D.; Coukos, G.; Crum, C.C.; Drapkin, R.; Etemadmoghadam, D.; et al. Rethinking ovarian cancer: Recommendations for improving outcomes. *Nat. Rev. Cancer* **2011**, *11*, 719–725. [CrossRef] [PubMed]

8. Heintz, A.P.M.; Odicino, F.; Maisonneuve, P.; Quinn, M.A.; Benedet, J.L.; Creasman, W.T.; Ngan, H.Y.S.; Pecorelli, S.; Beller, U. Carcinoma of the Ovary. *Int. J. Gynecol. Obstet.* **2006**, *95*, S161–S192. [CrossRef]

9. Kobayashi, H.; Yamada, Y.; Sado, T.; Sakata, M.; Yoshida, S.; Kawaguchi, R.; Kanayama, S.; Shigetomi, H.; Haruta, S.; Tsuji, Y.; et al. A randomized study of screening for ovarian cancer: A multicenter study in Japan. *Int. J. Gynecol. Cancer* **2008**, *18*, 414–420. [CrossRef] [PubMed]

10. Buys, S.S. Effect of Screening on Ovarian Cancer Mortality. *JAMA* **2011**, *305*, 2295. [CrossRef] [PubMed]

11. Jacobs, I.J.; Menon, U.; Ryan, A.; Gentry-Maharaj, A.; Burnell, M.; Kalsi, J.K.; Amso, N.N.; Apostolidou, S.; Benjamin, E.; Cruickshank, D.; et al. Ovarian cancer screening and mortality in the UK Collaborative Trial of Ovarian Cancer Screening (UKCTOCS): A randomised controlled trial. *Lancet* **2016**, *387*, 945–956. [CrossRef]

12. Paulsen, T.; Kjaerheim, K.; Kaern, J.; Tretli, S.; Tropé, C. Improved short-term survival for advanced ovarian, tubal, and peritoneal cancer patients operated at teaching hospitals. *Int. J. Gynecol. Cancer* **2006**, *16*, 11–17. [CrossRef] [PubMed]

13. Engelen, M.J.; Kos, H.E.; Willemse, P.H.; Aalders, J.G.; de Vries, E.G.; Schaapveld, M.; Otter, R.; van der Zee, A.G. Surgery by consultant gynecologic oncologists improves survival in patients with ovarian carcinoma. *Cancer* **2006**, *106*, 589–598. [CrossRef] [PubMed]

14. Earle, C.C.; Schrag, D.; Neville, B.A.; Yabroff, K.R.; Topor, M.; Fahey, A.; Trimble, E.L.; Bodurka, D.C.; Bristow, R.E.; Carney, M.; et al. Effect of surgeon specialty on processes of care and outcomes for ovarian cancer patients. *J. Natl. Cancer Inst.* **2006**, *98*, 172–180. [CrossRef] [PubMed]
15. Woo, Y.L.; Kyrgiou, M.; Bryant, A.; Everett, T.; Dickinson, H.O. Centralisation of services for gynaecological cancer—A Cochrane Systematic Review. *Gynecol. Oncol.* **2012**, *126*, 286–290. [CrossRef] [PubMed]
16. Valentin, L.; Hagen, B.; Tingulstad, S.; Eik-Nes, S. Comparison of "pattern recognition" and logistic regression models for discrimination between benign and malignant pelvic masses: A prospective cross validation. *Ultrasound Obstet. Gynecol.* **2001**, *18*, 357–365. [CrossRef] [PubMed]
17. Timmerman, D. The use of mathematical models to evaluate pelvic masses; can they beat an expert operator? *Best Pract. Res. Clin. Obstet. Gynaecol.* **2004**, *18*, 91–104. [CrossRef] [PubMed]
18. Meys, E.M.; Kaijser, J.; Kruitwagen, R.F.; Slangen, B.F.; van Calster, B.; Aertgeerts, B.; Verbakel, J.Y.; Timmerman, D.; van Gorp, T. Subjective assessment versus ultrasound models to diagnose ovarian cancer: A systematic review and meta-analysis. *Eur. J. Cancer* **2016**, *58*, 17–29. [CrossRef] [PubMed]
19. Timmerman, D.; Valentin, L.; Bourne, T.; Collins, W.P.; Verrelst, H.; Vergote, I. Terms, definitions and measurements to describe the sonographic features of adnexal tumors: A consensus opinion from the International Ovarian Tumor Analysis (IOTA) group. *Ultrasound Obstet. Gynecol.* **2000**, *16*, 500–505. [CrossRef] [PubMed]
20. Timmerman, D.; Testa, A.C.; Bourne, T.; Ameye, L.; Jurkovic, D.; van Holsbeke, C.; Paladini, D.; van Calster, B.; Vergote, I.; van Huffel, S.; et al. Simple ultrasound-based rules for the diagnosis of ovarian cancer. *Ultrasound Obstet. Gynecol.* **2008**, *31*, 681–690. [CrossRef] [PubMed]
21. Royal College of Obstetricians and Gynaecologists. *Management of Suspected Ovarian Masses in Premenopausal Women*; Green-top Guideline No. 62; Royal College of Obstetricians and Gynaecologists: London, UK, 2011.
22. The American College of Obstetricians and Gynecologists. Practice bulletin—Evaluation and Management of Adnexal Masses. *Obstet. Gynecol.* **2016**, *128*, e210–e226.
23. Kaijser, J.; Sayasneh, A.; van Hoorde, K.; Ghaem-Maghami, S.; Bourne, T.; Timmerman, D.; van Calster, B. Presurgical diagnosis of adnexal tumours using mathematical models and scoring systems: A systematic review and meta-analysis. *Hum. Reprod. Update* **2014**, *20*, 449–462. [CrossRef] [PubMed]
24. Timmerman, D.; van Calster, B.; Testa, A.; Savelli, L.; Fischerova, D.; Froyman, W.; Wynants, L.; van Holsbeke, C.; Epstein, E.; Franchi, D.; et al. Predicting the risk of malignancy in adnexal masses based on the Simple Rules from the International Ovarian Tumor Analysis group. *Am. J. Obstet. Gynecol.* **2016**, *214*, 424–437. [CrossRef] [PubMed]
25. Van Calster, B.; van Hoorde, K.; Valentin, L.; Testa, A.C.; Fischerova, D.; van Holsbeke, C.; Savelli, L.; Franchi, D.; Epstein, E.; Kaijser, J.; et al. International Ovarian Tumour Analysis, G. Evaluating the risk of ovarian cancer before surgery using the ADNEX model to differentiate between benign, borderline, early and advanced stage invasive, and secondary metastatic tumours: Prospective multicentre diagnostic study. *BMJ* **2014**, *349*, g5920. [CrossRef] [PubMed]
26. Meys, E.M.; Jeelof, L.S.; Achten, N.M.; Slangen, B.F.; Lambrechts, S.; Kruitwagen, R.F.; van Gorp, T. Estimating the risk of malignancy in adnexal masses: An external validation of the ADNEX model and comparison with other frequently used ultrasound methods. *Ultrasound Obstet. Gynecol.* **2016**. [CrossRef] [PubMed]
27. Sayasneh, A.; Ferrara, L.; de Cock, B.; Saso, S.; Al-Memar, M.; Johnson, S.; Kaijser, J.; Carvalho, J.; Husicka, R.; Smith, A.; et al. Evaluating the risk of ovarian cancer before surgery using the ADNEX model: A multicentre external validation study. *Br. J. Cancer* **2016**, *115*, 542–548. [CrossRef] [PubMed]
28. Szubert, S.; Wojtowicz, A.; Moszynski, R.; Zywica, P.; Dyczkowski, K.; Stachowiak, A.; Sajdak, S.; Szpurek, D.; Alcazar, J.L. External validation of the IOTA ADNEX model performed by two independent gynecologic centers. *Gynecol. Oncol.* **2016**, *142*, 490–495. [CrossRef] [PubMed]
29. Araujo, K.G.; Jales, R.M.; Pereira, P.N.; Yoshida, A.; de Angelo Andrade, L.; Sarian, L.O.; Derchain, S. Performance of the IOTA ADNEX model in the preoperative discrimination of adnexal masses in a gynecologic oncology center. *Ultrasound Obstet. Gynecol.* **2016**. [CrossRef]
30. Joyeux, E.; Miras, T.; Masquin, I.; Duglet, P.E.; Astruc, K.; Douvier, S. Before surgery predictability of malignant ovarian tumors based on ADNEX model and its use in clinical practice. *Gynecol. Obstet. Fertil.* **2016**, *44*, 557–564. [CrossRef] [PubMed]

31. Testa, A.; Kaijser, J.; Wynants, L.; Fischerova, D.; van Holsbeke, C.; Franchi, D.; Savelli, L.; Epstein, E.; Czekierdowski, A.; Guerriero, S.; et al. Strategies to diagnose ovarian cancer: New evidence from phase 3 of the multicentre international IOTA study. *Br. J. Cancer* **2014**, *111*, 680–688. [CrossRef] [PubMed]

32. DeLong, E.R.; DeLong, D.M.; Clarke-Pearson, D.L. Comparing the areas under two or more correlated receiver operating characteristic curves: A nonparametric approach. *Biometrics* **1988**, *44*, 837–845. [CrossRef] [PubMed]

33. Wilson, E.B. Probable inference, the law of succession, and statistical inference. *J. Am. Stat. Assoc.* **1927**, *22*, 209–212. [CrossRef]

34. Collins, G.S.; Reitsma, J.B.; Altman, D.G.; Moons, K.G. Transparent reporting of a multivariable prediction model for individual prognosis or diagnosis (TRIPOD): The TRIPOD statement. *BMJ* **2015**, *350*, g7594. [CrossRef] [PubMed]

35. Hartman, C.A.; Juliato, C.R.; Sarian, L.O.; Toledo, M.C.; Jales, R.M.; Morais, S.S.; Pitta, D.D.; Marussi, E.F.; Derchain, S. Ultrasound criteria and CA 125 as predictive variables of ovarian cancer in women with adnexal tumors. *Ultrasound Obstet. Gynecol.* **2012**, *40*, 360–366. [CrossRef] [PubMed]

36. Alcazar, J.L.; Pascual, M.A.; Olartecoechea, B.; Graupera, B.; Auba, M.; Ajossa, S.; Hereter, L.; Julve, R.; Gaston, B.; Peddes, C.; et al. IOTA simple rules for discriminating between benign and malignant adnexal masses: Prospective external validation. *Ultrasound Obstet. Gynecol.* **2013**, *42*, 467–471. [CrossRef] [PubMed]

37. Sayasneh, A.; Wynants, L.; Preisler, J.; Kaijser, J.; Johnson, S.; Stalder, C.; Husicka, R.; Abdallah, Y.; Raslan, F.; Drought, A.; et al. Multicentre external validation of IOTA prediction models and RMI by operators with varied training. *Br. J. Cancer* **2013**, *108*, 2448–2454. [CrossRef] [PubMed]

38. Nunes, N.; Ambler, G.; Foo, X.; Naftalin, J.; Widschwendter, M.; Jurkovic, D. Use of IOTA simple rules for diagnosis of ovarian cancer: Meta-analysis. *Ultrasound Obstet. Gynecol.* **2014**, *44*, 503–514. [CrossRef] [PubMed]

39. Tinnangwattana, D.; Vichak-ururote, L.; Tontivuthikul, P.; Charoenratana, C.; Lerthiranwong, T.; Tongsong, T. IOTA Simple Rules in Differentiating between Benign and Malignant Adnexal Masses by Non-expert Examiners. *Asian Pac. J. Cancer Prev.* **2015**, *16*, 3835–3838. [CrossRef] [PubMed]

40. Ruiz de Gauna, B.; Rodriguez, D.; Olartecoechea, B.; Auba, M.; Jurado, M.; Gomez Roig, M.D.; Alcazar, J.L. Diagnostic performance of IOTA simple rules for adnexal masses classification: A comparison between two centers with different ovarian cancer prevalence. *Eur. J. Obstet. Gynecol. Reprod. Biol.* **2015**, *191*, 10–14. [CrossRef] [PubMed]

41. Knafel, A.; Banas, T.; Nocun, A.; Wiechec, M.; Jach, R.; Ludwin, A.; Kabzinska-Turek, M.; Pietrus, M.; Pitynski, K. The Prospective External Validation of International Ovarian Tumor Analysis (IOTA) Simple Rules in the Hands of Level I and II Examiners. *Ultraschall Med.* **2015**, *37*, 516–523. [CrossRef] [PubMed]

42. Shih, I.-M.; Kurman, R. Ovarian Tumorigenesis—A Proposed Model Based on Morphological and Molecular Genetic Analysis. *Am. J. Pathol.* **2004**, *164*, 1511–1518. [CrossRef]

43. Valentin, L.; Ameye, L.; Jurkovic, D.; Metzger, U.; Lecuru, F.; van Huffel, S.; Timmerman, D. Which extrauterine pelvic masses are difficult to correctly classify as benign or malignant on the basis of ultrasound findings and is there a way of making a correct diagnosis? *Ultrasound Obstet. Gynecol.* **2006**, *27*, 438–444. [CrossRef] [PubMed]

44. Valentin, L.; Ameye, L.; Savelli, L.; Fruscio, R.; Leone, F.P.; Czekierdowski, A.; Lissoni, A.A.; Fischerova, D.; Guerriero, S.; van Holsbeke, C.; et al. Adnexal masses difficult to classify as benign or malignant using subjective assessment of gray-scale and Doppler ultrasound findings: Logistic regression models do not help. *Ultrasound Obstet. Gynecol.* **2011**, *38*, 456–465. [CrossRef] [PubMed]

45. Vergote, I.; Amant, F.; Ameye, L.; Timmerman, D. Screening for ovarian carcinoma: Not quite there yet. *Lancet Oncol.* **2009**, *10*, 308–309. [CrossRef]

46. Fischerova, D.; Zikan, M.; Dundr, P.; Cibula, D. Diagnosis, treatment, and follow-up of borderline ovarian tumors. *Oncologist* **2012**, *17*, 1515–1533. [CrossRef] [PubMed]

47. Vergote, I.; de Brabander, J.; Fyles, A.; Bertelsen, K.; Einhorn, N.; Sevelda, P.; Gore, M.; Kaern, J.; Verrelst, H.; Sjövall, K.; et al. Prognostic importance of degree of differentiation and cyst rupture in stage I invasive epithelial ovarian carcinoma. *Lancet* **2001**, *357*, 176–182. [CrossRef]

48. Ledermann, J.A.; Raja, F.A.; Fotopoulou, C.; Gonzalez-Martin, A.; Colombo, N.; Sessa, C.; Group, E.G.W. Newly diagnosed and relapsed epithelial ovarian carcinoma: ESMO Clinical Practice Guidelines for diagnosis, treatment and follow-up. *Ann. Oncol.* **2013**, *24* (Suppl. S6), vi24–vi32. [CrossRef] [PubMed]

49. Kurman, R.J.; Shih, I.-M. Molecular pathogenesis and extraovarian origin of epithelial ovarian cancer—Shifting the paradigm. *Hum. Pathol.* **2011**, *42*, 918–931. [CrossRef] [PubMed]
50. Amant, F.; Verheecke, M.; Wlodarska, I.; Dehaspe, L.; Brady, P.; Brison, N.; van Den Bogaert, K.; Dierickx, D.; Vandecaveye, V.; Tousseyn, T.; et al. Presymptomatic Identification of Cancers in Pregnant Women During Noninvasive Prenatal Testing. *JAMA Oncol.* **2015**, *1*, 814–819. [CrossRef] [PubMed]
51. Vanderstichele, A.; Busschaert, P.; Smeets, D.; Landolfo, C.; van Nieuwenhuysen, E.; Leunen, K.; Neven, P.; Amant, F.; Mahner, S.; Braicu, E.I.; et al. Chromosomal Instability in Cell-Free DNA as a Highly Specific Biomarker for Detection of Ovarian Cancer in Women with Adnexal Masses. *Clin. Cancer Res.* **2016**. [CrossRef] [PubMed]

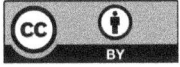

MDPI AG

St. Alban-Anlage 66

4052 Basel, Switzerland

Tel. +41 61 683 77 34

Fax +41 61 302 89 18

http://www.mdpi.com

Diagnostics Editorial Office

E-mail: diagnostics@mdpi.com

http://www.mdpi.com/journal/diagnostics

* 9 7 8 3 0 3 8 4 2 7 1